ESSENTIALS IN CYTOPATHOLOGY

Dorothy L. Rosenthal, MD, FIAC, Series Editor

Editorial Board

Syed Z. Ali, MD
Douglas P. Clark, MD
Yener S. Erozan, MD

W0051312

For further volumes:
http://www.springer.com/series/6996

Ricardo H. Bardales
Editor

Cytology of the Mediastinum and Gut Via Endoscopic Ultrasound-Guided Aspiration

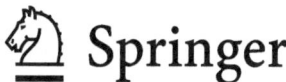 Springer

Editor
Ricardo H. Bardales
Pathology and Cytopathology
Outpatient Pathology Associates
Sacramento
California
USA

ISSN 1574-9053   ISSN 1574-9061 (electronic)
Essentials in Cytopathology
ISBN 978-3-319-12795-8   ISBN 978-3-319-12796-5 (eBook)
DOI 10.1007/978-3-319-12796-5

Library of Congress Control Number: 2014958743

Springer Cham Heidelberg New York Dordrecht London

Printed on acid-free paper

Springer is part of Springer Science+Business Media (www.springer.com)

TO: Waldetrudis, my beloved mother and best teacher, who patiently taught me the value of education.

Angela, Angie, and Ricky for their constant encouragement, support, and tolerance.

My mentors Abel Mejia, Benjamin Koziner, Leopold G. Koss, Klaus Schreiber, Norwin Becker, and Michael W. Stanley.

My pathology residents and cytology fellows.

Preface

Minimally invasive procedures for material procurement, such as fine-needle aspiration (FNA), are important for rapid, cost-effective, and accurate sampling and diagnosis of deep-seated masses. Thus, management of patients with such masses, particularly those with high-risk conditions, has been improved by the use of FNA. Obtaining samples from masses located around the midline such as the mediastinum, including lymph nodes for cancer staging, or small masses located in the wall of the gut is notoriously difficult or impossible by FNA under percutaneous ultrasound (US) guidance. The combination of endoscopic (E) or endorectal (ER) fiberoptic devices and radiological techniques, particularly US, has facilitated the procurement of material from such masses. EUS- and ERUS-guided FNA via transesophageal or transrectal approaches are the techniques of choice to sample such masses.

This book provides a comprehensive review of the EUS-FNA cytology of disease processes of the mediastinum and mediastinal lymph nodes with emphasis on lung and esophageal nodal cancer staging. The EUS-FNA cytology of intramural masses of the esophageal and gastrointestinal tract using a pattern-based diagnostic approach as well as ERUS-FNA cytology of intra- and extramural masses of the colorectum are also covered. Familiarity with the cytomorphology of "contaminating" normal luminal gastrointestinal contents obtained by EUS-FNA is emphasized, as the cytopathologist must be familiar with this pattern not often seen in the material obtained by percutaneous FNA approach. Technical considerations pertaining to the operator performing the procedure as well as to the cytopathologist, with emphasis on rapid onsite interpretation, are also covered.

In summary, the readers will find this book to be a useful practical guide for the cytological interpretation and differential diagnosis of lesions obtained by EUS-FNA of the mediastinum and gut and ERUS-FNA of the colorectum. All chapters are written by experts with many years of experience in the field of cytology and gastroenterology, and contain the cytology, histopathology, immuno-profile, molecular profile, and US features of the masses described. Numerous cytology and EUS images complement the text.

R. H. Bardales

Acknowledgements

My special thanks to the pathology residents and fellows at Hennepin County Medical Center, Minneapolis, who throughout the years have contributed with cases that always occupy special places in the library of my desk, brain, and most importantly, my heart. I also thank Mrs. Connie Walsh and Mr. Michael F. Griffin, developmental editors for Springer, and Richard Hruska, senior editor for Springer, for their constant support and patience. Special thanks to Mr. Rick M. Tracy, digital imaging specialist, Pathology Photography & Computer Graphic Department at the Johns Hopkins hospital, who made the photographs in Chap. 6 suitable for publication. Last but not the least, my special gratitude and admiration to Mrs. Elisabeth Lanzl, senior editor at the University of Chicago, for her undaunted efforts, despite my repetitive mistakes, to improve the English grammar and syntax of my manuscripts to transform them into readable documents. I have learnt so much from her in the past 25 years, and there are still lots of room for improvement.

Ricardo H. Bardales, MD, MIAC, ECNU

Contents

Contents

Contents

Contents

Contributors

Ricardo H. Bardales Pathology and Cytopathology, Outpatient Pathology Associates, Sacramento, CA, USA

Luis E. De Las Casas Department of Pathology, The University of Toledo Medical Center, Toledo, OH, USA

Zahra Maleki Department of Pathology, Division of Cytopathology, The Johns Hopkins Hospital, Baltimore, MD, USA

Shawn Mallery Division of Gastroenterology, Hepatology and Nutrition, Department of Internal Medicine, University of Minnesota, Minneapolis, MN, USA

Ali Nawras Department of Medicine/Gastroenterology, University of Toledo Medical Center, Toledo, OH, USA

Chapter 1
General Considerations of EUS and EUS-FNA

Ricardo H. Bardales

Endoscopic ultrasonography (EUS) uses the technology of endoscopy to introduce high-frequency ultrasound probes into the upper or lower part of the gastrointestinal (GI) tract to visualize its wall and adjacent structures. EUS identifies and evaluates lesions occurring in the wall of the GI tract, in periluminal (mediastinal, abdominal, and pelvic) lymph nodes, pancreas, the left side of the liver, the spleen, left kidney, left adrenal gland, and at times masses in the most medial parts of lung. EUS is a highly accurate clinical test for the detection, staging, and optimal management of esophageal, gastric, colorectal, pancreatic, and biliary tumors as well as the evaluation of thick gastric folds and benign pancreatic disease.

In the last two decades, EUS-guided fine-needle aspiration (FNA) has empowered EUS as a tool that provides a cytologic diagnosis, being definitive and therapy-guiding for primary tumors such as pancreatic adenocarcinoma and for cancer staging, i.e., in the lung, pancreas, stomach, and esophagus. EUS-FNA changes the therapeutic strategy in up to 15 and 30 % of patients with clinical suspicion of upper GI tract and pancreatic malignancy, respectively. The information provided by EUS-FNA prevents

R. H. Bardales (✉)
Pathology and Cytopathology, Outpatient Pathology Associates,
7750 College Town Drive Suite 102, Sacramento, CA 95826, USA

R. H. Bardales (ed.), *Cytology of the Mediastinum and Gut Via Endoscopic Ultrasound-Guided Aspiration,* Essentials in Cytopathology 25,
DOI 10.1007/978-3-319-12796-5_1,
© Springer International Publishing Switzerland 2015

unnecessary surgery in 30% of patients who have a primary malignancy. In addition, EUS-FNA is minimally invasive, relatively inexpensive, and associated with low risk of complications. Thus, EUS-FNA has become a diagnostic strategy of choice for masses in such sites. Furthermore, EUS and EUS-FNA may prove to be valuable diagnostic modalities that change clinical management in selected critically ill patients in the intensive care unit; transient intraprocedural complications were reported in 9% of interventions (6 of 63), predominantly related to brief oxygen desaturation. EUS and EUS-FNA have been proved useful in children as young as 5 years old with pancreas and mediastinal masses and when tissue was needed; the procedure is performed under general anesthesia and endotracheal intubation.

EUS-FNA provides an excellent sampling of lymph nodes, pancreatic tumors, and hepatic or left adrenal gland metastases. The overall sensitivity of EUS-FNA varies from 76 to 91%, the specificity from 84 to 100%, and the accuracy from 78 to 94%. Statistical analysis of 5667 EUS-FNAs of various targets showed a specificity of 92.8% (false positive rate 7.2%, 27/377 cases with cytohistological correlation) due to epithelial cell contamination, EUS sampling error, and cytology misdiagnosis; scenarios included lymph node sampling in the setting of Barrett's esophagus with dysplasia or early cancer, pancreas mass in chronic or autoimmune pancreatitis, reactive gastropathy, and nodal sampling for rectal cancer staging; EUS-FNA samples may be contaminated with cellular elements carried over during transmural needle passage resulting in diagnostic difficulties. Recent analysis shows a pooled sensitivity of 85% in the EUS-FNA of solid pancreatic masses. Cystic pancreatic lesions have a diagnostic rate of 66% with the use of EchoBrush. Less favorable results are seen for EUS-FNA of cystic lesions of the pancreas (54% sensitivity and 93% specificity) and GI wall masses. Still, the overall accuracy of EUS-FNA in patients with mural masses, who had previously failed endoscopic standard forceps biopsy procedures, is 81%. The nondiagnostic rate of EUS-FNA of pancreas is wide, ranging from 2 to 48%; factors will be further discussed in Chap. 2.

The overall risk of complications from EUS-FNA is low (1.6%), slightly higher than that for standard EUS alone; however, it appears acceptable. Perforation and aspiration pneumonia are rare. Acute extraluminal hemorrhage at the site of the aspiration occurs in 1.3% of patients; however, this is typically self-limited. Complications that may occur after the procedure include (but are not limited to) pancreatitis and infection. Aspiration of cystic pancreatic lesions conveys a 14% risk of infection, bleeding, or pancreatitis. Life-threatening mediastinitis has been reported after EUS-FNA of a mediastinal bronchogenic cyst. Therefore, antibiotic prophylaxis for patients with cysts and necrotic lesions after EUS-FNA is currently recommended by the American Society for Gastrointestinal Endoscopy (ASGE). However, prophylactic administration of antibiotics to prevent endocarditis is currently not recommended.

The incidence of needle-track tumor seeding in malignancies evaluated by EUS-FNA is difficult to assess, because surgical excision often removes the needle pathway or the tumor responds to chemotherapy. Peritoneal implants have been reported in 1 of 46 patients (2.2%) and 7 of 43 patients (16%) when EUS-FNA or percutaneous-guided FNA was used, respectively, for the initial diagnosis of nonmetastatic pancreatic carcinoma.

New applications for EUS are also emerging, including interventional EUS. The basic principle is to advance a needle under EUS guidance into a target in the vicinity of the gut to inject an agent, drain fluid, or form a fistula. EUS-guided celiac plexus block is one of the procedures to prevent or control the intractable pain in patients with pancreas cancer. Local delivery of chemotherapy is another application in constant development. The most successful procedure is cyst or pseudocyst drainage under EUS guidance, which has become the standard of care. Drainage of pelvic abscesses of various sizes has been successfully done with no complications. EUS-guided transgastric or transduodenal cholangiopancreatography has been reported useful and with few complications in patients with obstructive jaundice when standard endoscopic retrograde cholangiopancreatography (ERCP) was unsuccessful. Therapeutic pancreas cyst alcohol ablation is being investigated and is an area of constant evolution that needs further evaluation. Placement of EUS-guided gold fiducial markers to be used as point of reference for image-guided radiation therapy in unresectable pancreatic adenocarcinoma has been done with promising results. Finally, radioactive seeds have been placed under EUS guidance and results are under evaluation to assess benefits.

Further Reading

Bardales RH, Stelow EB, et al. Review of endoscopic ultrasound-guided fine-needle aspiration cytology. Diagn Cytopathol. 2006;34(2):140–75.

Berzosa M, Davies SF, et al. Diagnostic bedside EUS in the intensive care unit: a single-center experience. Gastrointest Endosc. 2013;77(2):200–8.

Das A, Chak A. Endoscopic ultrasonography. Endoscopy. 2004;36(1):17–22.

Hawes RH. The evolution of endoscopic ultrasound: improved imaging, higher accuracy for fine needle aspiration and the reality of endoscopic ultrasound-guided interventions. Curr Opin Gastroenterol. 2010;26(5):436–44.

Hewitt MJ, McPhail MJ, et al. EUS-guided FNA for diagnosis of solid pancreatic neoplasms: a meta-analysis. Gastrointest Endosc. 2012;75(2):319–31.

Gleeson FC, Kipp BR, et al. False positive endoscopic ultrasound fine needle aspiration cytology: incidence and risk factors. Gut. 2010;59(5):586–593.

Jhala NC, Jhala DN, et al. Endoscopic ultrasound-guided fine-needle aspiration. A cytopathologist's perspective. Am J Clin Pathol. 2003;120(3):351–67.

Lozano MD, Subtil JC, et al. EchoBrush may be superior to standard EUS-guided FNA in the evaluation of cystic lesions of the pancreas: preliminary experience. Cancer Cytopathol. 2011;119(3):209–14.

Thornton GD, McPhail MJ, et al. Endoscopic ultrasound guided fine needle aspiration for the diagnosis of pancreatic cystic neoplasms: a meta-analysis. Pancreatology. 2013;13(1):48–57.

Chapter 2
Technical Considerations of EUS and EUS-FNA

Ricardo H. Bardales, Luis E. De Las Casas, Ali Nawras and Shawn Mallery

Echoendoscopes

Echoendoscopes have a transducer mounted in front of the optic lens and are available in two different designs, radial and curvilinear, depending on the orientation of the transducer (Figs. 2.1, 2.2).

R. H. Bardales (✉)
Pathology and Cytopathology, Outpatient Pathology Associates, 7750 College Town Drive Suite 102, Sacramento, CA 95826, USA
e-mail: rhbardales@aol.com

L. E. De Las Casas
Department of Pathology, The University of Toledo Medical Center, Hospital Bldg., Room 0136G Mail Stop 1068, 3000 Arlington Avenue, Toledo, OH 43614, USA
e-mail: luis.delascasas@utoledo.edu

A. Nawras
Department of Medicine/Gastroenterology, University of Toledo Medical Center, 3000 Arlington Ave, Mail Stop 1186, Toledo, OH 43614, USA
e-mail: ali.nawras@utoledo.edu

S. Mallery
Division of Gastroenterology, Hepatology and Nutrition, Department of Internal Medicine, University of Minnesota, MMC 36, 420 Delaware St. SE, Minneapolis, MN 55455, USA
e-mail: malle004@umn.edu

R. H. Bardales (ed.), *Cytology of the Mediastinum and Gut Via Endoscopic Ultrasound-Guided Aspiration,* Essentials in Cytopathology 25, DOI 10.1007/978-3-319-12796-5_2,
© Springer International Publishing Switzerland 2015

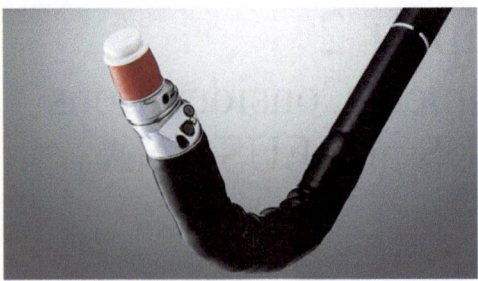

FIG. 2.1. Echoendoscope with radial transducer. (Olympus GF-UE 160, Olympus America, Center Valley, PA)

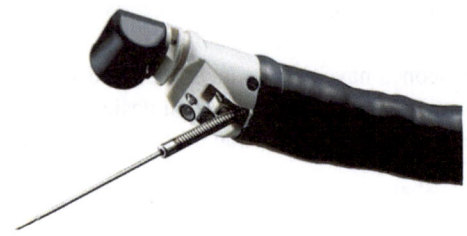

FIG. 2.2. Echoendoscope with linear transducer. (Olympus GF-UC140P, Olympus America, Center Valley, PA)

A radial scanning echoendoscope produces a 360° real-time view perpendicular to the shaft of the echoendoscope (Fig. 2.3). A linear-array instrument produces a real-time, sector-shaped image parallel to the shaft of the echoendoscope (Figs. 2.4, 2.5). This imaging plane with the linear instrument allows for visualization of the entire length of a needle, which is advanced through the working channel of the echoendoscope whereas a radial device only displays a cross-section of the needle (a small spot) where the needle crosses the imaging plane (Fig. 2.3b). For this reason, virtually all endoscopic ultrasound fine-needle aspiration (EUS-FNA) is performed using linear-array instruments. For colorectal EUS, rigid probes for the rectum and flexible forward-viewing echocolonoscopes are available. Doppler (color) ultrasound allows for visualization of blood flow in vascular structures. Acoustic contact of the ultrasound (US) probe and the wall of the gastrointestinal (GI) tract are typically obtained through a water-filled balloon that surrounds

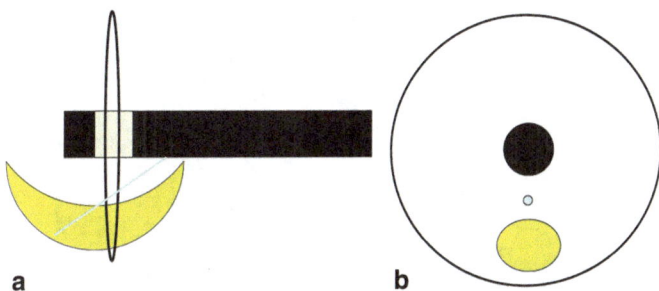

FIG. 2.3. A radial scanning echoendoscope produces a 360° real-time view perpendicular to the shaft of the echoendoscope (*B* shows expected ultrasound image with scope positioned as in *A*)

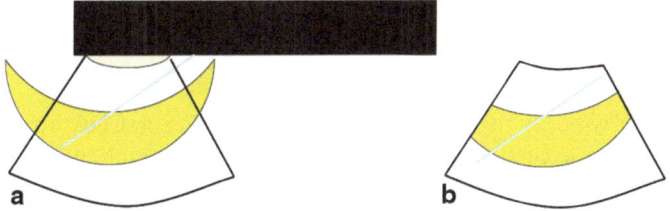

FIG. 2.4. A linear-array instrument, the preferred choice for fine-needle aspiration (*FNA*), produces a sector-shaped image in a plane parallel to the endoscope. This allows visualization of the entire length of a needle, which has been advanced into the banana

the probe or less frequently by filling the GI lumen with water. Samples can be obtained effectively from small lesions irrespective of the organ affected. Tumors <5 mm in diameter can be detected and sampled by the use of high-resolution echoendoscopes.

Needle Type and Caliber

Several manufacturers, including Wilson-Cook, Boston Scientific, Olympus, and Medi-Globe, produce commercially available specialized needle assemblies for use with EUS. Our gastroenterology

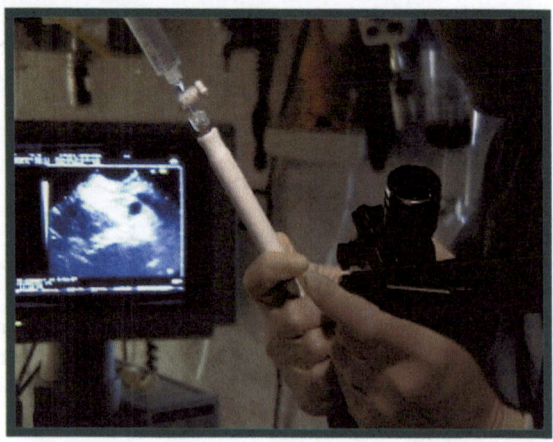

FIG. 2.5.   The real-time image is visualized on a sector-shaped sound field on a computer monitor

team typically uses 19-, 22-, and 25-gauge Wilson-Cook needles with an excursion of up to 8 cm beyond the distal end of the 125-cm-long echoendoscope. A 25-gauge needle is routinely used for the sampling of most lesions and produces sufficient quantities of minimally bloody specimens. When needed, a 19-gauge needle is used for obtaining tissue fragments from suspected stromal tumors and for performing immunohistochemical (IHC) stains in cell-block slides. About 22- and 19-gauge needles may be used for draining of fluid collections and sampling of mediastinal lymph nodes with sclerosis. Ancillary studies for lymphoma work-up are performed successfully in aspirates, with use of a 25-gauge needle. The use of a 19-gauge Trucut needle may result in more frequent complications (i.e., infection and bleeding) and may not increase the accuracy, particularly when mediastinal lesions are evaluated; however, the approach does appear safe and accurate for the sampling of intestinal wall and abdominal masses.

Role of the Endosonographer

EUS identification, staging, and FNA, particularly of pancreatic masses, are technically challenging and require special training. Accuracy is operator dependent and correlates with experience. EUS competence is difficult to achieve even for advanced endoscopy trainees. The current recommendation of the American Society for Gastrointestinal Endoscopy (ASGE) for EUS competence is 150 EUS procedures; however, this number may not be sufficient and most trainees may require 250 or more. Factors that influence this variable rate include cognitive and technical skills of the operator and station/organ examined, i.e., esophagogastric versus pancreatobiliary imaging; other factors are availability of cases in the trainer center and continuous access to perform EUS exams. Ideally, EUS-FNA competence starts once EUS competence is reached. EUS-FNA sampling accuracy has been shown to increase from 33 to 91% following a 2-month period of formal mentored training. The ASGE recommends a minimum of supervised 50 EUS-FNA procedures, 25–30 of which should be aimed to pancreas masses to reach the level of competence. The ASGE recommendation of 25–30 supervised EUS-FNA procedures for the diagnosis of pancreatic adenocarcinoma is supported by a study showing that there was a significant increase in the sensitivity of EUS-FNA diagnosis of pancreatic cancer, which plateaued at 80–90% after 30 procedures. EUS-FNA cytology interpretation errors during the initial learning phase are primarily due to inadequate specimens.

The Aspiration Technique

The needle selection should be based on the physical characteristics and anatomic location of the target lesion.

a) Solid lesions

One of the basic principles of aspiration of solid lesions is that the thicker the needle is and the more negative pressure applied, the more bloody and diluted the sample can be. Therefore for most cases, the tendency is to use one of the smallest caliber needles available: a 25-gauge needle.

A 25-gauge needle is usually initially utilized in most solid lesions. It is better to have the stylet in place completely occluding the needle lumen until the target lesion is reached. Having the stylet occluding the needle lumen before reaching the target tumor avoids carryover of nonlesion material/contaminants. These contaminants include gastrointestinal mucosal epithelial fragments, fluids from the lumen, or any tissue fragments form organs trespassed with the needle before reaching the tumor. These nondiagnostic elements cause marked dispersion of the diagnostic material, which gets diluted, swollen, and blurred by fluid or widely scattered between numerous non-lesional tissue fragments making it more difficult to interpret.

Once the stylet is completely removed, it is more useful to do the aspiration without suction (the cellular material gets in the needle lumen by the action of capillary forces due to the fast movement of the needle within the lesion). The use of a 25-gauge needle allows the operator to have a "feel" of the consistency of the lesion. On occasions when there is no too much physical distance to move the needle within the lesion or when after the first pass a very hard lesion is felt, application of negative pressure with a syringe is recommended.

When the needle is in the lesion, it is recommended to move it back and forth as fast as possible within the target lesion. Keeping the needle still or longer than 5–10 seconds (depending on Doppler examination) within the lesion often causes the specimen to clot or be too bloody resulting in "sausages" of blood and fibrin obscuring the diagnostic elements, which are difficult to smear onto a glass slide and interpret on cytological rapid on-site interpretation. When clotting occurs, attempts to make smears should be avoided and the material should be placed in fixative and submitted to the pathology laboratory to be processed as a cell block.

The consistency of the lesion felt by the operator who is moving the needle is also important in deciding the next step. For example, in gastric wall lesions, a soft consistency generally narrows the differential diagnosis to lipomas, neuroendocrine tumors , or heterotopic pancreatic tissue. Gastrointestinal stromal tumors (GISTs), Schwannomas, and leiomyomas are generally firm rather than soft.

Solid masses for practical purposes could be approached in three ways based on their consistency: hard, gritty or rubbery, and soft.

Hard masses: Most of these lesions are associated with a very fibrotic or desmoplastic stroma. In these cases, the lesion "grabs" the needle and it is difficult to move the needle within the lesion; not uncommonly the needle gets bent because of the attempts to move the needle fast. The best approach is to use a 22- or a 19-gauge needle and perform the FNA applying suction. The smears are generally not very cellular but are often diagnostic. Several passes might be required. It is advised to try as much as possible to sample different areas of the mass when diagnostic material is not obtained with the first attempt. The use of a 19-gauge needle is recommended when GIST is suspected to obtain material for a cell-block preparation and perform immunostains and molecular tests in the paraffin-embedded material.

Gritty or rubbery masses: These lesions could be sampled using a 25-gauge needle, with or without suction. The movement of the needle within the lesion has to be as fast as the size and location of the tumor allow it. Generally, 1–3 passes provide enough diagnostic material. It is important to keep in mind that when additional studies might be required (e.g., metastatic carcinoma of unknown origin, metastatic lung adenocarcinomas where epidermal growth factor receptor (EGFR) testing might be requested, metastatic colorectal cancer where *KRAS* gene mutations are often needed, etc.), additional passes up to the discretion of the cytopathologist and interventional gastroenterologist are often required.

Soft masses: These lesions are usually sampled with a 25-gauge needle without suction. After the first pass when the tumor type is identified, subsequent passes are triaged according to the ancillary test required (e.g., flow cytometry for lymphomas or cell-block material for immunostains).

b) Cystic lesions

The larger, stiffer, and more awkward 19-gauge needle is reserved for aspirating/draining larger cysts as it allows for a faster procedure and the aspiration of viscous contents. It may also be used for obtaining tissue fragments from the cyst wall.

Some needles come with a stylet whose tip is beveled to the needle tip whereas others come with a protruding ball-tip stylet. The ball-tip version might protect the endoscope channel should the needle be deployed accidently. In general, the ball-tip stylet must be withdrawn by about 1 cm before puncture in order to "sharpen" the needle. Following puncture, the stylet is pushed in to extrude any plugs of extraneous tissue. A prospective trial comparing FNA with and without stylet tried to answer the question of whether the use of the stylet is needed or not. The general conclusion was to use the stylet during the first pass and do the others without stylet. In our practice, we still use the stylet for all passes.

It is paramount to remember that the use of thinner needle, less dwelling time in vascular lesions, and no or minimal suction yields less bloody but diagnostic samples.

Number of Passes

In general, the number of passes is inversely proportional to the experience of the endosonographer and the presence of the cytopathologist during the procedure. Without a cytopathologist in attendance, 5–7 passes should be made for pancreatic masses and miscellaneous lesions, 3–5 for lymph nodes, and 2–3 for liver metastases to ensure a high degree of certainty for making a correct diagnosis (80 % sensitivity and 100 % specificity). However, these guidelines in preference to rapid on-site smear evaluation are associated with a 10–15 % reduction in diagnostic accuracy, extra procedure time, increased risk, and need for an increased number of needles, at considerable expense. We must emphasize that rapid on-site evaluation of adequacy is a better means of assessing the number of passes needed to obtain diagnostic material than is adherence to a set number of needle passes.

Role of the Cytopathologist

EUS-FNA cytology interpretation requires a high level of communication and trust between the endosonographer and the cytopathologist. The clinical and imaging data provided by the endosonographer are paramount for the cytopathologist final diagnosis. The cytopathologist should know the route that the needle travels to be aware of possible carryover of contaminants at the time of microscopic evaluation of the sample. Ultimately, it is the cytopathologist's role to tell the endosonographer when to end lesion sampling. This interaction is highly beneficial for patient management.

Specimen Handling

Briefly, the step-by-step procedure is as follows:

1. The sample is deposited on a glass slide by the endosonographer. The use of the stylet or air flushing is recommended if the sample is from a solid lesion. If the sample is from a cystic lesion, use the stylet to deposit the first few drops and make smears (one DiffQuik®for rapid interpretation and one ethanol-fixed for later stain) or use liquid-based cytology solution. If the needle gets clogged with blood clot, use the stylet and place the material in a glass slide and then transfer it to a container with formalin for cell-block processing; do not attempt to make smears.
2. Visible tissue fragments are separated from the blood, "picked up" with the edge of another glass slide, and smeared onto one or more slides. This results in a concentrated specimen that can be examined immediately under the microscope for on-site evaluation.
3. Air-dried smears fixed with methanol are stained with the DiffQuik® stain for immediate reading; 95 % ethanol-fixed smears are stained with the Papanicolaou or H&E stain for later reading. One smear for each staining per pass is usually prepared.
4. Rapid on-site evaluation of the DiffQuik®-stained smear for specimen adequacy and preliminary diagnosis is encouraged.

5. Let the remainder of the bloody sample clot on the glass slide. Submit the blood clot in formalin for cell-block processing. The methodology is the same as for FNA of masses in superficial organs.
6. Additional passes are requested if indicated for additional purposes, i.e., cell block, cell marker analysis, ultrastructural studies, cytogenetics, cultures for infectious agents, molecular techniques, and research protocols.

Rapid On-Site Evaluation

Rapid on-site smear evaluation (ROSE) by the cytopathologist optimizes the EUS-FNA diagnostic accuracy and minimizes the technique's insufficiency rate (i.e., sampling failure and poor handling/preparation of aspirated material), resulting in a reduced likelihood of complications for the patient. Thus, it is recommended that a cytotechnologist or cytopathologist be in attendance for all aspiration procedures to assess specimen adequacy and give a preliminary diagnosis which, in many instances, is the definitive diagnosis (Fig. 2.6).

ROSE increases the diagnostic yield and sensitivity to near or higher than 90 %, and the specificity and positive predictive values to near 100 %. However, it requires special training and can be time-consuming. A preliminary diagnosis may guide further clinical investigation or treatment, and it may determine whether ancillary studies are needed for a more specific diagnosis. It appears that lesion characteristics, aspiration site, or tumor type do not significantly influence the diagnostic results. Negative or nondiagnostic EUS-FNA interpretation requires correlation with clinical and/or imaging findings for a decision on further appropriate management. In general, it has been shown that a reduction in rate of nondiagnostic specimens is observed when ROSE is performed; however, the range of this rate is broad (as low as 2–36 % and higher).

Other factors that influence diagnostic yield include experience of the gastroenterologist, number of passes, and sample processing. It has been suggested that when EUS-FNAs of pancreas masses are performed by experienced endosonographers, ROSE may not

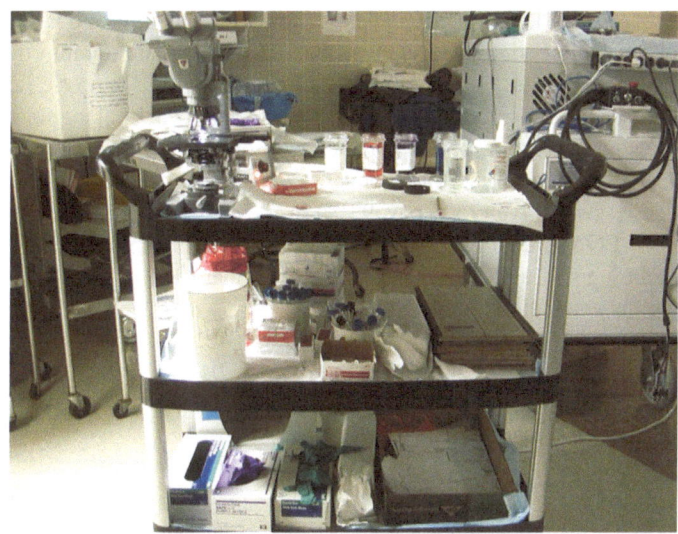

FIG. 2.6. A cart with needed equipment for rapid reading stain and sample triaging should be kept in the endoscopy suite. Rapid on-site smear evaluation by the cytopathologist optimizes the EUS-FNA diagnostic accuracy

offer benefit in reducing the nondiagnostic rate when rinse of the sample is placed in liquid-based solution for later slide preparation and interpretation. This prospective comparative study with and without ROSE showed similar diagnostic and nondiagnostic rates of around 75 and 25%, respectively. We prefer conventional smear preparation and encourage the use of ROSE.

Final and not less important is the fact that ROSE by a cytopathologist is often not cost-effective and henceforth not provided due to limited resources—a window for the controversial use of liquid-based cytology in EUS-FNA of solid masses.

Liquid-Based Cytology

The preferred method of EUS-FNA cytology sample preparation and evaluation is conventional smears stained with Romanowsky and Papanicolaou or H&E stains. The use of liquid-based cytology (LBC) requires a familiarity with the interpretation of this type of specimens. Clear cytological detail due to better fixation and lack of obscuring blood or air drying artifact are factors that may improve diagnostic yield. Reports suggest improvement of diagnostic rate and sensitivity with the use of LBC as reported in cholangiopancreatography-guided FNA of pancreas. However, others report that LBC is less accurate than conventional smears (81 versus 95 %) and less sensitive (75 versus 93 %) in the evaluation of pancreatic EUS-FNA, predominantly of solid masses without an on-site cytopathologist. Less controversial is the fact that LBC may be useful for the evaluation of cystic lesions.

Further Reading

Alsohaibani F, Girgis S, et al. Does onsite cytotechnology evaluation improve the accuracy of endoscopic ultrasound-guided fine-needle aspiration biopsy? Can J Gastroenterol. 2009;23(1):26–30.

Bardales RH, Stelow EB, et al. Review of endoscopic ultrasound-guided fine-needle aspiration cytology. Diagn Cytopathol. 2006;34(2):140–75.

Berzosa M, Davies SF, et al. Diagnostic bedside EUS in the intensive care unit: a single-center experience. Gastrointest Endosc. 2013;77(2):200–8.

Cermak TS, Wang B, et al. Does on-site adequacy evaluation reduce the nondiagnostic rate in endoscopic ultrasound-guided fine-needle aspiration of pancreatic lesions? Cancer Cytopathol. 2012;120(5):319–25.

Das A, Chak A. Endoscopic ultrasonography. Endoscopy. 2004;36(1):17–22.

Eltoum IA, Chhieng DC, et al. Cumulative sum procedure in evaluation of EUS-guided FNA cytology: the learning curve and diagnostic performance beyond sensitivity and specificity. Cytopathology. 2007;18(3):143–50.

Jhala NC, Jhala DN, et al. Endoscopic ultrasound-guided fine-needle aspiration. a cytopathologist's perspective. Am J Clin Pathol. 2003;120(3):351–67.

LeBlanc JK, Ciaccia D, et al. Optimal number of EUS-guided fine needle passes needed to obtain a correct diagnosis. Gastrointest Endosc. 2004;59(4):475–81.

Lee JK, Choi ER, et al. A prospective comparison of liquid-based cytology and traditional smear cytology in pancreatic endoscopic ultrasound-guided fine needle aspiration. Acta Cytol. 2011;55(5):401–7.

Mertz H, Gautam S. The learning curve for EUS-guided FNA of pancreatic cancer. Gastrointest Endosc. 2004;59(1):33–7.

Siddiqui MT, Gokaslan ST, et al. Split sample comparison of ThinPrep and conventional smears in endoscopic retrograde cholangiopancreatography-guided pancreatic fine-needle aspirations. Diagn Cytopathol. 2005;32(2):70–5.

Skov BG, Baandrup U, et al. Cytopathologic diagnoses of fine-needle aspirations from endoscopic ultrasound of the mediastinum: reproducibility of the diagnoses and representativeness of aspirates from lymph nodes. Cancer. 2007;111(4):234–41.

Stelow EB, Bardales RH, et al. Pitfalls in endoscopic ultrasound-guided fine-needle aspiration and how to avoid them. Adv Anat Pathol. 2005;12(2):62–73.

Varadarajulu S, Fraig M, et al. Comparison of EUS-guided 19-gauge Trucut needle biopsy with EUS-guided fine-needle aspiration. Endoscopy. 2004;36(5):397–401.

Wani S, Cote GA, et al. Learning curves for EUS by using cumulative sum analysis: implications for American Society for Gastrointestinal Endoscopy recommendations for training. Gastrointest Endosc. 2013;77(4):558–65.

Chapter 3
EUS-FNA of Mediastinal Masses

Ricardo H. Bardales and Shawn Mallery

The mediastinum is arbitrarily divided into superior, anterior, middle, and posterior compartments. The topographic mediastinal location of a mass is important for elaborating a differential diagnosis, i.e., superior mediastinum (thymoma, thymic cyst, thyroid, parathyroid, lymph nodes), anterior (thymoma, thymic cyst, germ cell tumors, thyroid, parathyroid, paraganglioma, hemangioma, lipoma, lymph nodes), middle (pericardial and bronchial cysts, lymph nodes), and posterior (gastroenteric cysts, neurogenic tumors, paraganglioma), because these masses have a predilection for a particular location over the others.

The most common isolated mediastinal abnormality is the lymph node enlargement of unknown etiology. The underlying process may be benign (i.e., sarcoidosis, tuberculosis, histoplasmosis) or malignant (i.e., metastatic cancer, lymphoma). Less commonly, a

R. H. Bardales (✉)
Outpatient Pathology Associates, Pathology and Cytopathology,
7750 College Town Drive Suite 102, Sacramento, CA 95826, USA
e-mail: rhbardales@aol.com

S. Mallery
Division of Gastroenterology, Hepatology and Nutrition, Department of
Internal Medicine, University of Minnesota, MMC 36,
420 Delaware St. SE, Minneapolis, MN 55455, USA

R. H. Bardales (ed.), *Cytology of the Mediastinum and Gut Via Endoscopic*   19
Ultrasound-Guided Aspiration, Essentials in Cytopathology 25,
DOI 10.1007/978-3-319-12796-5_3,
© Springer International Publishing Switzerland 2015

primary benign or malignant mediastinal mass may be the cause of a mediastinal abnormality. Some of these lesions, particularly those located in the anterior and middle compartments, can be evaluated successfully by fine-needle aspiration (FNA) by use of an endoscopic ultrasound (EUS) or endobronchial ultrasound (EBUS) approach, avoiding a more aggressive technique. Mediastinoscopy or transtracheal biopsy can also provide access to the superior and anterior mediastinum and gives a pathologic diagnosis; however, these approaches may carry significant morbidity and cost. Recent studies show that EUS-FNA and EBUS-FNA are the most cost-effective and minimally invasive nonsurgical techniques for the study of the mediastinum. EBUS-FNA is not covered in this book.

EUS and EUS-FNA are minimally invasive diagnostic modalities that in experienced hands yield sensitivity and specificity in the range of 80–90 % in the evaluation of mediastinal masses and lymph nodes. EUS and EUS-FNA have access to paratracheal lymph nodes and lesions located in the posterior and inferior mediastinum. EBUS and EBUS-FNA have access to pretracheal masses and those adjacent to main bronchi particularly in the right side. Only those masses pertaining to the mediastinum and sampled by EUS-FNA are described in this chapter. Lymph node sampling for cancer staging is detailed in Chap. 4.

The presence of contaminating esophagogastric luminal contents may limit or prevent an adequate cytological interpretation and is further discussed in Chap. 5. Rapid onsite evaluation of the specimen by an experienced cytopathologist is paramount to assess specimen adequacy, triage the sample (i.e., cultures, immunophenotype in lymphoma, immunostains, cytogenetics, and molecular tests for possible targeted therapy in malignancies), and improve the diagnostic accuracy of the test.

Retrosternal Goiter

Occasionally, EUS-FNA is used for the evaluation of a retrosternal mass. Although EUS findings are suspicious for retrosternal goiter, finding bland-appearing follicular epithelial cells, colloid,

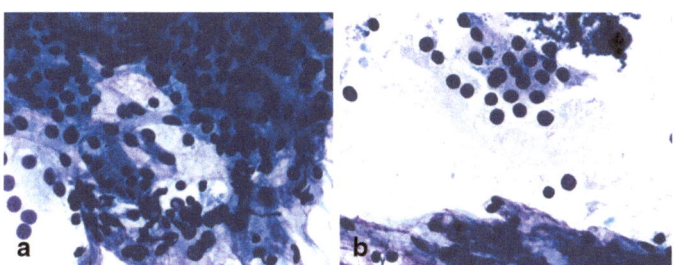

FIG. 3.1   Substernal goiter. Sheets of bland-appearing follicular epithelial cells and colloid (**a**). Focal oxyphilic change is also present (**b**). (DiffQuik stain, high magnification)

and variable numbers of macrophages in the EUS-FNA smears will confirm a benign diagnosis, often corresponding to a benign thyroid nodule as seen in nodular hyperplasia. The cytologic criteria for diagnosing neoplastic and nonneoplastic thyroid conditions and their differential diagnoses are similar to those described in thyroid cytology books (Fig. 3.1a, b).

Thymoma

Thymoma is a neoplasm of thymic epithelial cells that occurs almost exclusively in adults. Familial forms are exceptional. Patients may be asymptomatic, have local thoracic manifestations of thoracic mass compression, or have a paraneoplastic syndrome, myasthenia gravis being the most common, or erythroid hyperplasia or aplasia among others. Myasthenia gravis is an autoimmune disease with circulating autoantibodies that bind to the nicotinic acetylcholine receptor (AChR) located in the subsynaptic membrane of the neuromuscular junction or motor end plate.

Histopathology Histologically, *thymomas* show an admixture of neoplastic epithelial cells and nonneoplastic lymphocytes in various proportions (Fig. 3.2a). The epithelial cells may be plump, stellate, or spindle-shaped. Invasion of the tumor beyond the capsule

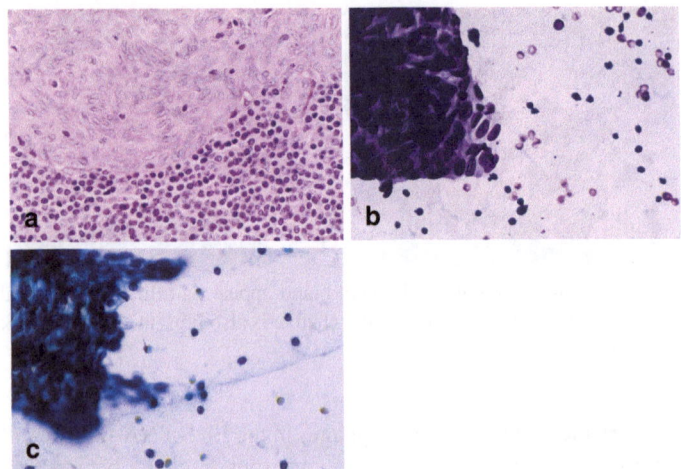

Fig. 3.2   Thymoma. Histology of a benign thymoma (**a**). Smears show cohesive elongated and epithelioid cells along with small lymphocytes and a background of proteinaceous fluid (**b**, **c**). (**a**, H&E stain intermediate magnification; **b**, **c**, DiffQuik and Papanicolaou stain, respectively, both high magnification)

is required for identification of the tumor as an *invasive thymoma*, which does not exhibit cytologic features of malignancy. The third type of thymic neoplasm is *thymic carcinoma*, which is rare, has a large variety of histologic patterns (epidermoid, sarcomatoid, clear-cell, basaloid, edenoid cystic, mucoepidermoid, papillary, anaplastic), has obvious cytologic features of malignancy, is rarely associated with myasthenia gravis, and, in contrast to thymomas shows neuroendocrine differentiation.

Immuno-Profile Epithelial cells are keratin, EMA, CEA, and p63 positive. Lymphocytes are of T-cell phenotype and express CD3 and CD4. TdT may be variably expressed. Co-expression of BCL2 and p53 is seen in most thymomas with a stronger reactivity in clinically aggressive tumors. Thymic carcinomas are CD5+, CD117+, CD70+ (member of the tumor necrosis factor family), and GLUT-1+; thymomas are rarely positive for these markers.

Molecular Profile Aberrations of chromosome 6 are common in thymomas, mostly in region 6q25.2. Thymic carcinomas show loss of 16q, 6, 3p, and 17p and gain of 1q, 17q, and 18.

FNA Findings Smears show variable cellularity and a characteristic dual population of epithelial and lymphoid cells. Epithelial cells may be tightly or loosely cohesive and round to polygonal or even spindle-shaped, simulating a mesenchymal neoplasm (Figs. 3.2b, c). Invasive thymomas have bland cytologic features, and the diagnosis is made histologically on the resected specimen. Thymic carcinomas have a malignant cytomorphology that may resemble nonepithelial tumors such as sarcoma.

EUS Features Imaging studies show a lobulated mass in the anterosuperior mediastinum that may be calcified. In a reported case of recurrent malignant thymoma (thymic carcinoma) diagnosed by EUS-guided trucut biopsy, the EUS demonstrated two hypoechoic heterogeneous masses with a focal, lobulated, and ill-defined edge, and measured 20×10 mm and 15×13 mm.

Rare Thymic Tumors

Neuroendocrine tumors, i.e., carcinoid, small-cell neuroendocrine carcinoma, and large-cell neuroendocrine carcinoma as well as stromal tumors, i.e., thymolipoma, and thymic stromal sarcoma, have been described.

Mediastinal Cysts

Thymic cysts are acquired or congenital. Acquired thymic cysts are usually large, multiloculated with attenuated thymic tissue, and relatively rare. Cytology smears show squamous cells, variable numbers of lymphocytes and red blood cells, and debris. Treatment is complete resection, and recurrence is rare. Congenital thymic cysts

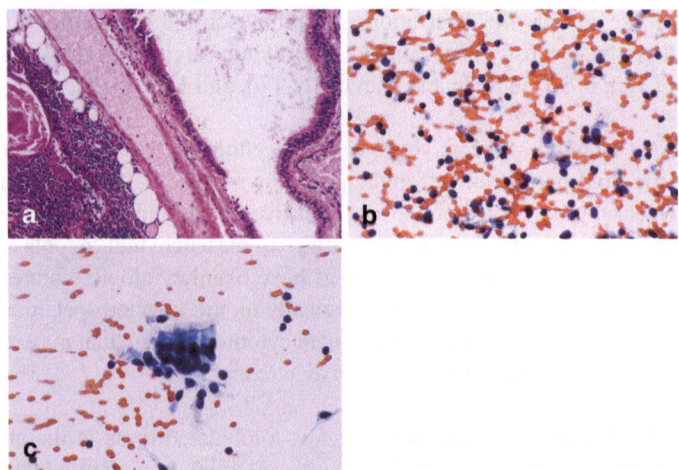

Fɪɢ. 3.3   Congenital thymic cyst. The epithelium is ciliated and lymphoid tissue is seen to the left side of frame (**a**). Smears show proteinaceous fluid, lymphocytes, and rare ciliated epithelial cells (**b, c**). (**a**, H&E stain, intermediate magnification; **b, c**, Papanicolaou and DiffQuik stain high magnification)

occuring in the first two decades of life are unilocular, have a thin wall lined with cuboidal or ciliated epithelium, and contain a clear fluid (Fig. 3.3a, b, c). Excision is curative.

Parathyroid cysts may be large and permeate between tissue planes extending to the superior mediastinum, are often not functioning, and aspirates show a water-like clear fluid and rare macrophages; measurement of parathyroid hormone levels in the cyst fluid (sample needs to be frozen immediately) will support the diagnosis.

Pericardial or celomic cysts are usually located at the right cardiophrenic angle, are unilocular, lined by a single mesothelial layer, and contain clear fluid.

Mediastinal *foregut cysts* account for ~20% of mediastinal masses and are congenital anomalies from a structure destined to become part of the trachea or bronchi (bronchial cysts) or esophagus, stomach, and intestine (esophageal, gastric, and enteric cysts, respectively). *Bronchial cysts* commonly occur along the tracheobronchial tree, often superior to the carina, but may be found in the wall of the esophagus. These contain inspissated mucus and are lined with ciliated epithelium, although squamous metaplasia may be focally present. *Esophageal cysts* are commonly intramural and are located in the lower third of the esophagus. The lining epithelium may be squamous, ciliated, columnar, or a combination. *Gastric and enteric cysts*, lined with gastric and intestinal type epithelium, respectively, are located attached to or within the wall of the esophagus and are often associated with vertebral malformations. EUS confirms the cystic nature of these lesions, and EUS-FNA shows ciliated, squamous, or glandular cells, depending on the cyst type (Fig. 3.4a). Acute mediastinitis is a rare complication therefore prophylactic antibiotic therapy is recommended following EUS-FNA of mediastinal cysts.

EUS Features of Mediastinal Cysts.

US characteristics are similar to those seen in cysts of other organs, including oval or round shape, marked hypoechogenicity, sharply defined margins, and posterior acoustic enhancement (Fig. 3.4b, c). Heterogeneity may be present in the presence of a dense fluid. An echogenic mass of variable size may be identified attached to the wall when a solid phase mural component is present; the solid component has variable vascularity on Doppler exam.

Adenopathy of Unknown Etiology

EUS-FNA can readily identify and sample lymph nodes in the subcarinal, paraesophageal, and paratracheal regions, but not in the pretracheal space or intrapulmonary regions. EUS-FNA is often performed for sonographically benign or suspicious lymph nodes when an abnormal finding will alter management.

Metastasis In patients with a history of extrathoracic malignancy, metastasis from such a source is the major cause of mediastinal

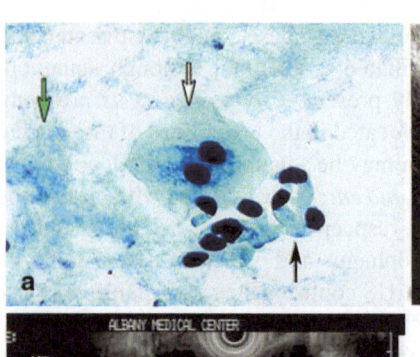
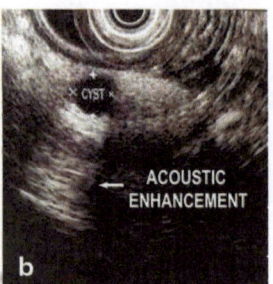
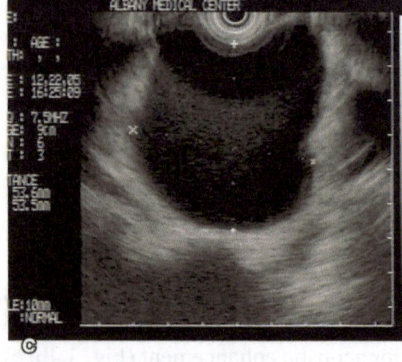

Fig. 3.4   EUS-FNA and EUS features of mediastinal cysts. Smears show columnar (*black solid arrow*), and/or ciliated, and/or squamous (*white arrow*) cells along with proteinaceous fluid (*red arrow*), debris, and mucus (**a**). Cysts are markedly hypoechoic/ anechoic, round or oval and show sharply demarcated borders and posterior acoustic enhancement (**b**, **c**, linear EUS). (**a**, Romanowsky stain, high magnification)

involvement, and as a result surgical diagnostic procedures are often not indicated. Renal-cell carcinoma is capable of metastasizing to the lungs or mediastinum years after diagnosis of the primary tumor. On the contrary, in patients without previous malignancy and mediastinal adenopathy, EUS-FNA identifies benign or malignant processes with equal proportion. When malignancy of unknown origin is diagnosed involving the mediastinal lymph nodes, a lung primary is subsequently identified in >80% of cases.

Infectious Lymphadenopathy It is the most frequently diagnosed cause of unexplained adenopathy by EUS-FNA in our experience (Midwest of USA), and *Mycobacteria* and *Histoplasma* are the most likely diagnoses. EUS-FNA alters the subsequent work-up and therapy in ~75% of such patients, obviating the need for more invasive diagnostic studies such as thoracotomy. EUS-FNA smears show lymphocytes, granulomas, and necrosis in varying proportions (Fig. 3.5a, b). Special stains for fungus (i.e., methenamine silver and PAS) and mycobacteria (i.e., acid-fast and Fite) performed in the smears or cell block provide information for initiation of appropriate therapy until confirmatory cultures are available. A negative direct stain neither excludes an infectious process nor confirms a noninfectious inflammatory etiology. Similarly, absence of granulomas and presence of granular amorphous material and crystals in the aspirate smear does not exclude a fungal infection; on the contrary, these findings are not uncommon in histoplasmosis (Fig. 3.6a, b). Thus, granulomas, lymphocytes, and necrosis must be taken in the context of the patient's clinical scenario, including geographic area of living. Large yeast forms with thick clear capsule and mucoid background are seen in *Cryptococcus* lymphadenitis, often seen in immunosuppressed individuals and often preceded by *Cryptococcus* meningitis (Fig. 3.7).

Sarcoidosis Sarcoidosis deserves special comment. It is identified in ~5% of mediastinal lymph nodes evaluated by EUS and sampled by EUS-FNA. The reported specificity and sensitivity of EUS-FNA in the diagnosis of sarcoidosis are 94 and 100%, respectively. The technique provides a useful alternative for the diagnosis of this condition. The smears are usually of limited cellularity and show cohesive epithelioid granulomas, cell degeneration, and often

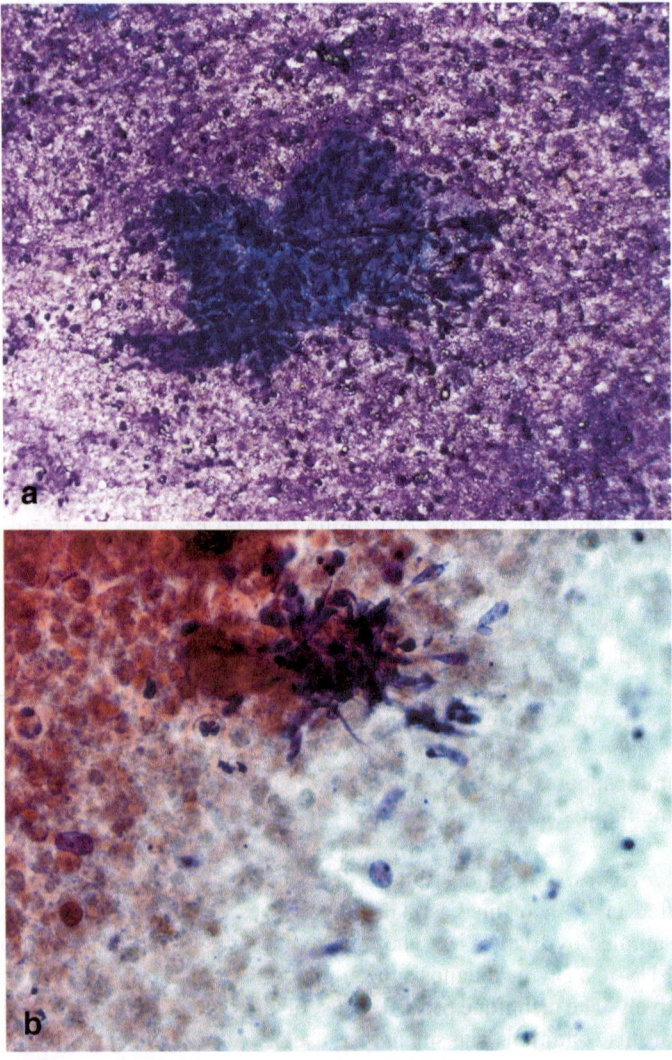

FIG. 3.5   Tuberculosis. Granulomas (**a**), rare single histiocytes nuclei (**b**), and granular necrotic background are seen in tuberculosis. Note the lack of acute inflammation or individual cell necrosis in the necrotic background. (**a**, DiffQuik stain intermediate magnification; **b**, Papanicolaou stain high magnification)

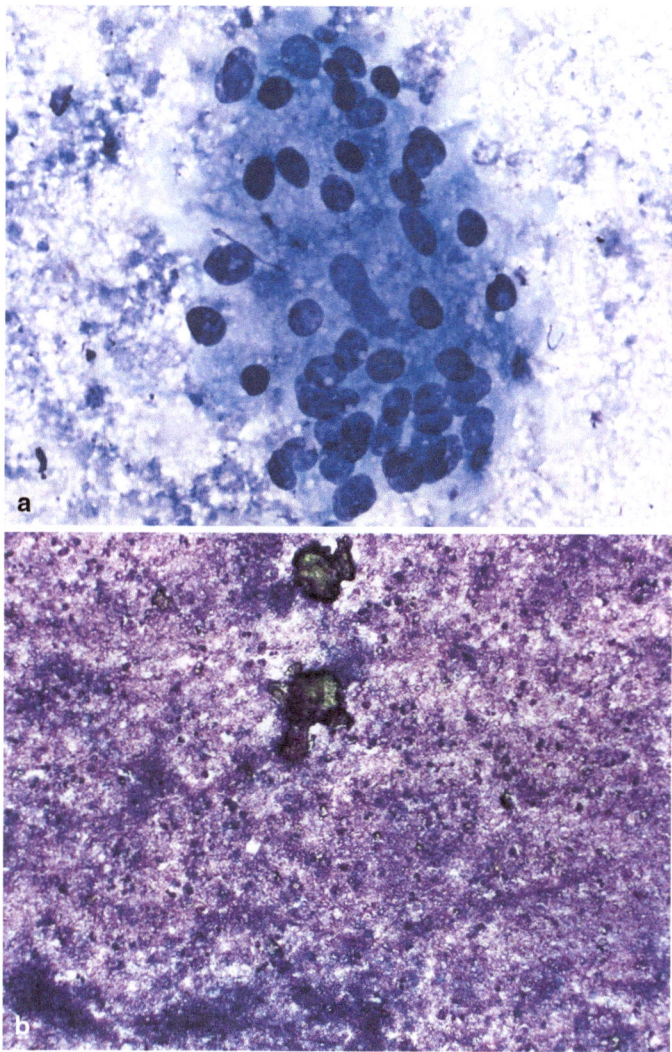

Fɪɢ. 3.6   Histoplasmosis. Multinucleated histiocytes (**a**), crystals (**b**) and granular necrotic background are not uncommonly seen in histoplasmosis. Silver stain for fungus in the smears was positive for fungal yeast organisms in this case. (**a, b** DiffQuik stain high and intermediate magnification)

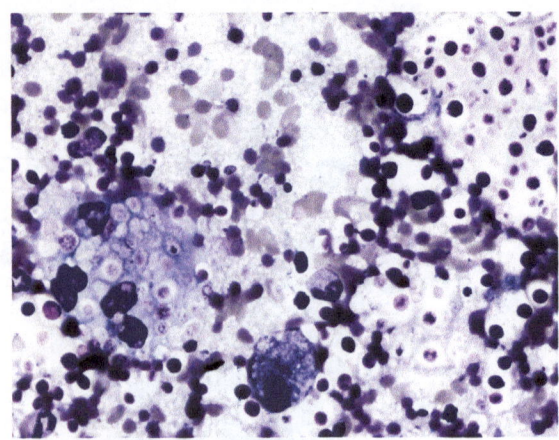

FIG. 3.7   Cryptococcal lymphadenitis. Note numerous round large yeast forms surrounded by a clear capsule in a mucoid background best seen in Romanowsky-stained smears. (DiffQuik stain, high magnification)

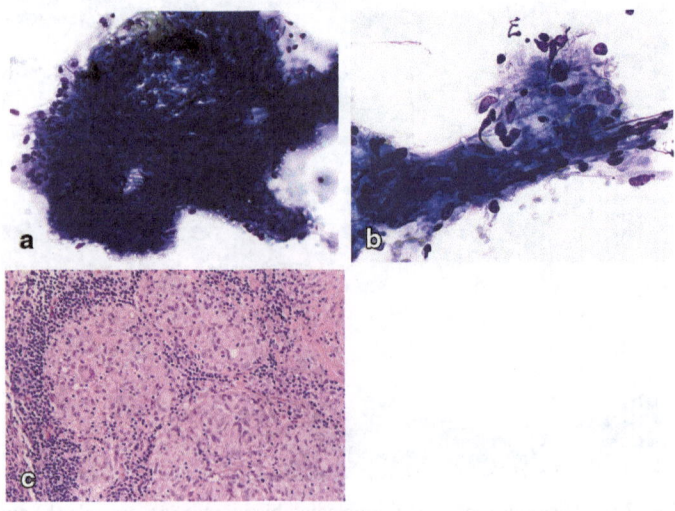

FIG. 3.8   Sarcoidosis. Tight granulomas with slight cell degeneration and often lack of necrosis (a–c) are characteristic of sarcoidosis. (a, b DiffQuik stain high magnification; c, H&E intermediate magnification)

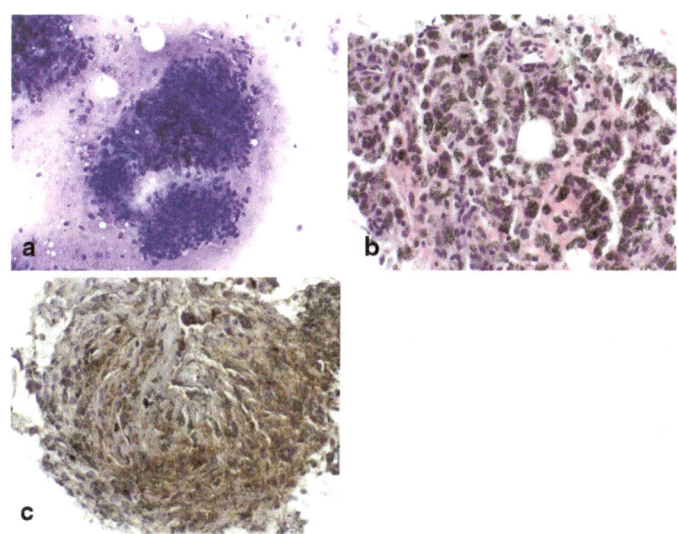

F_IG. 3.9   Anthracosilicotic spindle cell pesudotumor. Poorly formed epithelioid granulomas with cytoplasmic pigment mimic a neoplastic process (**a, b**). Immunostain for MAC387 (macrophage marker) is positive (**c**). In addition, evaluation under polarized light helps in the diagnosis. (**a**, DiffQuik stain intermediate magnification; **b**, Cell block H&E stain high magnification; **c**, Immunoperoxidase stain high magnification)

lack necrosis (Fig. 3.8a, b, c). Cultures for fungi and mycobacteria are negative. Core biopsy may be particularly useful in this setting.

Anthracotic and Anthracosilicotic Spindle-Cell Pseudotumors, the result of a phenotypic transformation of histiocytes into spindle cells caused by the foreign dust silica are rare reactive spindle-cell proliferations that may involve mediastinal lymph nodes and can mimic neoplastic processes clinically, radiologically, and pathologically. The differential diagnosis includes spindle-cell melanoma, inflammatory pseudotumor, Kaposi's sarcoma, and mycobacterial pseudotumor. The clinical history, bland cytomorphology, positivity under polarized-light examination, and positive immunoreactivity with histiocytic markers (CD68, MAC387) are important for the diagnosis of anthracosilicotic spindle-cell pseudotumor (Fig. 3.9a, b, c).

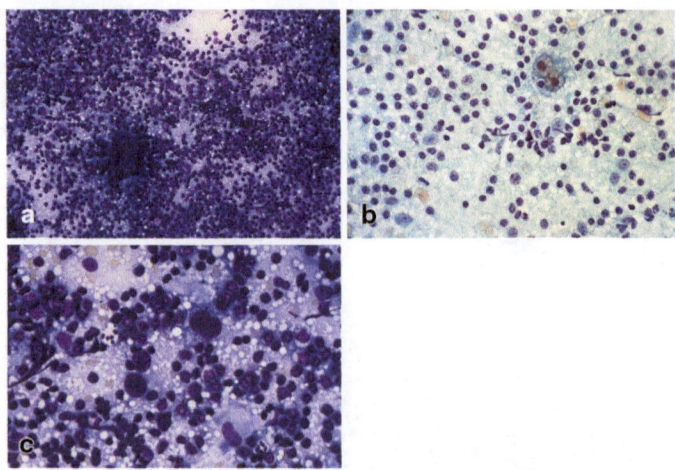

Fɪɢ. 3.10   Hodgkin lymphoma. The smears show a population of poly-morphous lymphoid cells; granulomas may be present (**a**). Reed-Sternberg cells (**b**) and variants (**c**) are present in such a background. (**a**, **c** DiffQuik intermediate and high magnification; **b**, Papanicolaou stain high magnification)

Malignant Lymphoma, the most common primary neoplasm of the mediastinum, can involve the anterior, superior, and middle compartments as a primary process or as a manifestation of disseminated disease. Hodgkin lymphoma and lymphoblastic and large-cell non-Hodgkin lymphoma are the most common varieties. Marginal-zone B-cell lymphoma involving the thymus, particularly in patients with Sjögren disease or rheumatoid arthritis, may be seen in rare instances.

Hodgkin Lymphoma This is the most common lymphoma of the mediastinum and can involve lymph nodes, the thymus, or both. The nodular sclerosing variant is the most common type and affects young and older adults, preferentially women. Cytology smears, in these cases show scant cellularity and significant cell degeneration. Variable numbers of plasma cells, eosinophils, histiocytes, and a polymorphous population of lymphocytes resembling reactive lymphoid hyperplasia or even granulomas mimicking a granu-

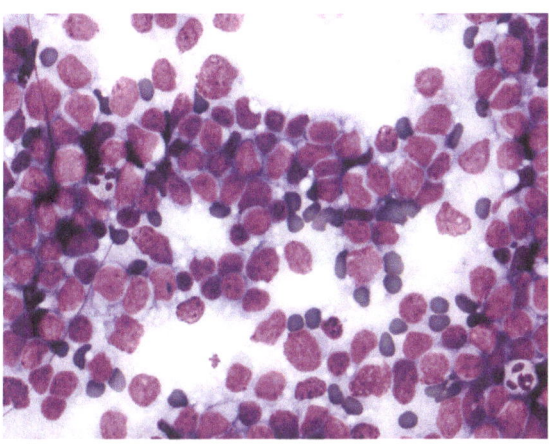

Fig. 3.11 Lymphoblastic lymphoma of the mediastinum. A monomorphous population of small to medium sized lymphoid cells with irregular nuclear contours and scattered mitoses is present. (DiffQuik stain, high magnification)

lomatous infection are also seen. Identification of Reed–Sternberg cells, their mononuclear variants, and lacunar cells is necessary for the diagnosis (Fig. 3.10a, b, c). The differential diagnosis includes anaplastic large-cell lymphoma and germ-cell tumors; however, in this latter diagnosis smears are more cellular, degree of anaplasia is greater, and the number of small lymphocytes is smaller than in Hodgkin's lymphoma. The syncytial variant of Hodgkin lymphoma exhibits loosely cohesive cells of various sizes that may mimic a metastatic deposit.

Lymphoblastic Lymphoma This tumor commonly involves the anterosuperior mediastinum, affects adolescents, predominantly males, and usually has an immature T-cell phenotype (WHO classification: precursor T-cell lymphoblastic lymphoma). Cytology smears show a monomorphic population of small atypical lymphoid cells with a convoluted nuclear membrane, numerous mitoses, and apoptotic nuclei (Fig. 3.11). The differential diagnosis includes neuroblastoma and also small lymphocytes from reactive

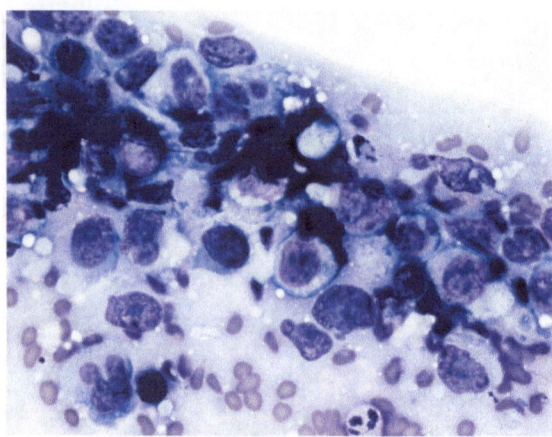

Fɪɢ. 3.12   Primary mediastinal lymphoma. This large cell type lymphoma often occurs in middle age women and mimics an epithelial malignancy and the syncytial variant of Hodgkin lymphoma. (DiffQuik stain high magnification)

lymphoid hyperplasia. However, neuroblastoma usually presents in the posterior mediastinum of young patients, and smears show rosettes and a fibrillary background. Lymphocyte-rich thymoma is also included in the differential diagnosis; however, lymphocytes lack atypia. Metastatic small-cell carcinoma, also in the differential diagnosis, presents in the mediastinum of adults who have a history of smoking and the smears show karyorrhexis, crushing artifact, and cell molding.

Primary Mediastinal Large B-Cell Lymphoma This lymphoma affects the thymus and/or lymph nodes of patients, preferentially women in the second and third decades of life, who frequently have superior vena cava syndrome. Smears show a monomorphic population of mostly dissociated large lymphoid cells with large irregular nuclei, and variable numbers of cell clusters, which can resemble a nonhematologic process (Fig. 3.12). In cases with significant sclerosis, cellularity is less optimal, and the atypical lymphoid cells may be damaged, making the diagnosis difficult. In this scenario, the differential diagnosis should include nodular scleros-

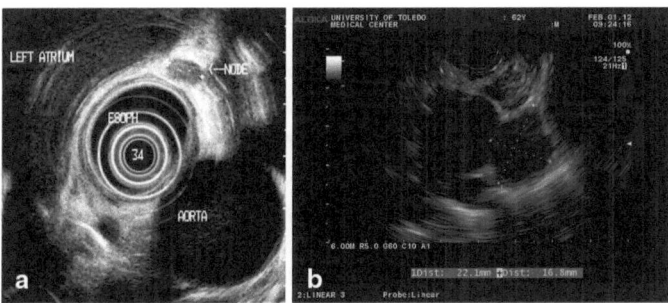

F IG . 3.13   EUS, benign lymph nodes. Ultrasound features of a benign lymph node include less hypoechogenicity than malignant lymph nodes, flat to oval shape, and poorly defined borders (**a**, radial EUS). Additional features include presence of hilum and hilar blood flow on Doppler exam. Ultrasound features of granulomatous lymphadenopathies may mimic malignancy; this case of sarcoidosis involving the aorto-pulmonary window lymph node shows prominent hypoechogenicity and irregular margins (**b**, linear EUS)

ing Hodgkin lymphoma. Primary mediastinal B-cell lymphoma expresses CD10 and BCL6, suggesting germinal-center-cell derivation and, in contrast to diffuse large B-cell lymphoma, rarely expresses BCL2. CD200 has recently been proposed as a useful marker with greater sensitivity (94 %) than CD23, MAL, and TRAF for distinguishing it from diffuse large B-cell lymphoma. The differential diagnosis also includes malignant thymoma, germ cell tumor, and the syncytial variant of Hodgkin lymphoma.

Ultrasound Features of Reactive and Infectious Lymph Nodes

Reactive lymph nodes usually have the following characteristics: hypoechogenicity, slightly ill-defined margins, hilum and hilar vascular pattern except lymph nodes <5 mm, lack of periph-

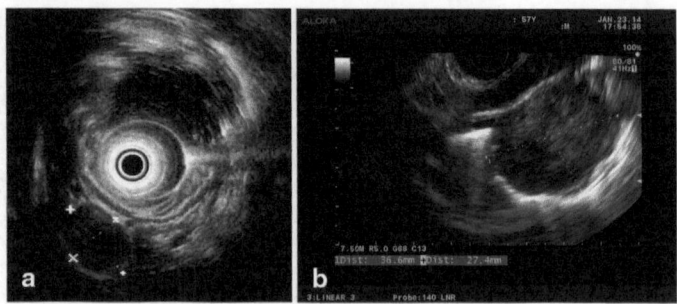

F<small>IG</small>. 3.14   EUS, malignant lymph node. Ultrasound features of a malignant lymph node include marked hypoechogenicity, round shape,
sharp borders, lack of hilum, and chaotic blood flow on Doppler exam
(**a**, radial). Marked hypoechogenicity and lobulated sharp margins are
seen in this large oddly-shaped metastatic paraesophageal lymph node
(**b**, linear)

eral blood flow by Doppler examination, and flat or oval shape
(Fig. 3.13a). Lymph nodes involved by granulomatous infectious processes including tuberculosis may have pronounced cystic necrosis and lymph node confluence that mimic malignancy
(Fig. 3.13b).

Ultrasound Features of Lymph Nodes Involved
by Metastases

Lymph nodes-affected by metastases are usually in the territory
of lymphatic drainage of the primary tumor, unless is a widely
metastatic process; and, the metastatic lymph node may be as
small as 0.5 cm. Lymph nodes often have the following characteristics: round, usually markedly hypoechogenic, absent hilum,
eccentric cortical hypertrophy, partial or total cystic necrosis,

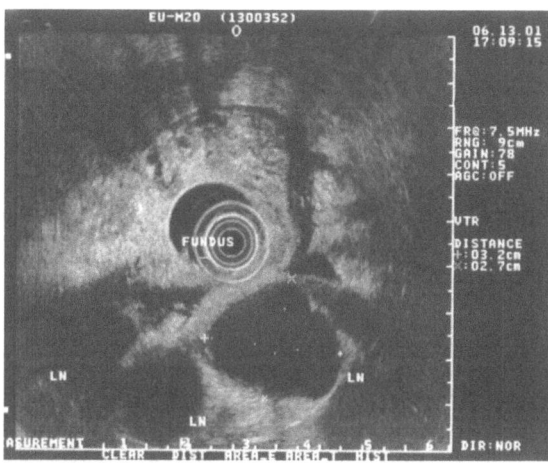

FIG. 3.15 Radial EUS, lymphoma. Large paragastric and mediastinal round and oval lymph nodes with marked hypoechogenicity and a pseudocystic appearance are seen in this case of large cell lymphoma

sharp margins, abnormal peripheral vascularization, and may be confluent (Fig. 3.14). The lymph node may be hyperechogenic with microcalcifcations in metastatic ovarian serous papillary carcinoma. The lymph node margins are ill-defined when there is lymph node extracapsular spread.

Ultrasound Features of Lymph Nodes Involved by Lymphomas

Lymph nodes are usually round or oval, markedly hypoechoic reticulated/micronodular, rarely necrotic, have sharp margins, and the hilum may be absent or present, usually with an exaggerated vascular pattern. Posterior acoustic enhancement may be present when there is marked hypoechogenicity ("pseudocystic" appearance) (Fig. 3.15)

Further Reading

Bardales RH, Stelow EB, et al. Review of endoscopic ultrasound-guided fine-needle aspiration cytology. Diagn Cytopathol. 2006;34(2):140–75.

Batsis C. Mediastinal lymphadenopathy: assessing clinical utility of EUS-FNA. Surg Endosc. 2011;25(8):2756–57.

Catalano MF, Rosenblatt ML, et al. Endoscopic ultrasound-guided fine needle aspiration in the diagnosis of mediastinal masses of unknown origin. Am J Gastroenterol. 2002;97(10):2559–65.

Cho CM, Al-Haddad M, et al. Rescue Endoscopic Ultrasound (EUS)-Guided trucut biopsy following suboptimal eus-guided fine needle aspiration for mediastinal lesions. Gut Liver. 2013;7(2):150–56.

Jhala NC, Jhala DN, et al. Endoscopic ultrasound-guided fine-needle aspiration. A cytopathologist's perspective. Am J Clin Pathol. 2003;120(3):351–67.

Larghi A, Rodriguez-Wulff E, et al. Recurrent malignant thymoma diagnosed by EUS-guided Trucut biopsy. Gastrointest Endosc. 2006;63(6):859–60.

Srinivasan R, Bhutani MS, et al. Clinical impact of EUS-FNA of mediastinal lymph nodes in patients with known or suspected lung cancer or mediastinal lymph nodes of unknown etiology. J Gastrointestin Liver Dis. 2012;21(2):145–52.

Stelow EB, Lai R, et al. Endoscopic ultrasound-guided fine-needle aspiration of lymph nodes: the hennepin county medical center experience. Diagn Cytopathol. 2004;30(5):301–06.

Wildi SM, Hoda RS, et al. Diagnosis of benign cysts of the mediastinum: the role and risks of EUS and FNA. Gastrointest Endosc. 2003;58(3):362–68.

Zeppa P, Barra E, et al. Impact of endoscopic ultrasound-guided fine needle aspiration (EUS-FNA) in lymph nodal and mediastinal lesions: a multicenter experience. Diagn Cytopathol. 2011;39(10):723–29.

Chapter 4
EUS and EUS-FNA in Lung, Esophageal, and Gastrointestinal Tract Nodal Cancer Staging

Ricardo H. Bardales and Shawn Mallery

Endoscopic ultrasound (EUS) is superior to cross-sectional imaging for the evaluation of local tumor (T) and mediastinal lymph nodes (LN) staging of lung and esophageal cancer, and T and LN staging in rectal cancer. EUS evaluation of mediastinum for nodal staging requires proper training in the form of lectures, observation, and supervised practice. Conversion of the conventional anatomy concept seen in static cross-sectional imaging to the real-life non-static one in EUS is one of the difficulties to master linear EUS.

Sonographic criteria may be used to assess the likelihood of metastasis within a visible lymph node (Fig. 4.1). These criteria are equally identifiable using radial or linear devices. Table 4.1 summarizes the sonographic criteria used for evaluation of nodal staging. If all four criteria are fulfilled, there is a 90 % possibility of malignancy. The presence of a single criterion indicates a low

R. H. Bardales (✉)
Pathology and Cytopathology, Outpatient Pathology Associates,
7750 College Town Drive Suite 102, Sacramento, CA 95826, USA
e-mail: rhbardales@aol.com

S. Mallery
Division of Gastroenterology, Hepatology and Nutrition,
Department of Internal Medicine, University of Minnesota,
MMC 36, 420 Delaware St. SE, Minneapolis, MN 55455, USA

R. H. Bardales (ed.), *Cytology of the Mediastinum and Gut Via Endoscopic*   39
Ultrasound-Guided Aspiration, Essentials in Cytopathology 25,
DOI 10.1007/978-3-319-12796-5_4,
© Springer International Publishing Switzerland 2015

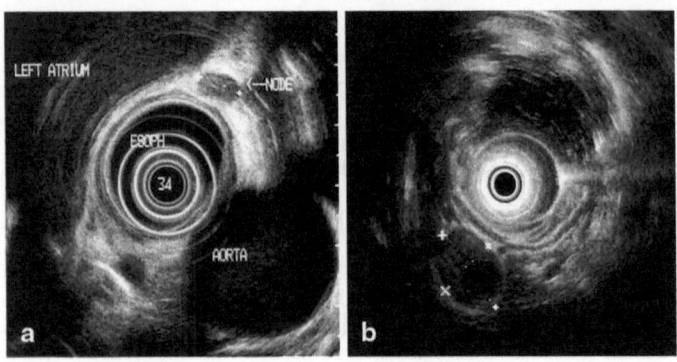

FIG. 4.1. Nodal cancer staging. Ultrasound features of benign (**a**) and suspicious (**b**, calipers) lymph nodes

TABLE 4.1. Nodal staging sonographic criteria (Fig. 4.1).

N0	Sonographic feature	N1
<1 cm	Size	>1 cm
Isoechoic/slightly hypoechoic, echogenic vascular hilum present, heterogenous echotexture	Echogenicity, hilum, vascularity	Hypoechoic, homogeneous echotexture, hilum absent, chaotic vascularity by Doppler examination
Oval, flat	Shape	Round
Indistinct	Demarcation	Sharp/infiltrating/lobulated

N0 negative, *N1* suspicious

possibility of malignancy. Needle aspiration, using a linear device, is used to confirm malignancy in sonographically equivocal nodes or when a definitive cytologic diagnosis alters management.

Lung Cancer

Evaluation of the mediastinum by EUS began in the early 1990s and has recently been expanded by the use of endobronchial ultrasound (EBUS) following the same principle applied to the bronchoscope. Thus, using different ports of access, both gastroenterologists and

Table 4.2. Abbreviated nodal non-small cell lung cancer staging. (AJCC Cancer Staging Manual. 7th ed. Springer. New York, 2010).

Regional lymph nodes (N)	
N1	Metastasis to ipsilateral peribronchial and/or ipsilateral hilar LNs, and intrapulmonary LNs including involvement by direct extension of the primary tumor
	Intrapulmonary LNs: hilar (proximal lobar), peribronchial, interlobar, lobar, and segmental
N2	Metastasis to ipsilateral mediastinal and/or subcarinal LNs
	Mediastinal LNs: paratracheal, pre- and retrotracheal (includes precarinal), aortic (includes aorto-pulmonary window, periaortic, ascending aortic, and phrenic), subcarinal, periesophageal, inferior pulmonary ligament
N3	Metastasis to contralateral (mediastinal, hilar, ipsilateral or contralateral scalene, or supraclavicular) LNs

LNs lymph nodes

pulmonologists evaluate the mediastinum in a complementary manner to perform an almost complete mediastinal nodal staging in an accurate, minimally invasive, and cost-effective approach. EUS findings impact patient management and surgery can be avoided in ~50% of the patients.

Direct tumor extension and nodal staging in lung cancer are paramount for deciding therapy options. Definitions of practical use for the cytopathologist assisting a nonsmall-cell lung cancer (NSCLC) staging are given in Table 4.2, which summarizes the American Joint Cancer Commission (AJCC) guidelines for lung cancer staging.

The cytopathologist needs to be aware that metastasis to subcarinal or ipsilateral mediastinal LN (N2) implies stage IIIA disease, while contralateral LN metastasis (N3) or direct mediastinal invasion (T3) implies stage IIIB disease and may prevent a patient from undergoing surgery (Fig. 4.2).

Computerized tomography (CT) scan is the standard imaging modality for lung cancer, but is poor at staging the mediastinum (sensitivity, 50–70%) and unreliable for detecting LNs < 1 cm. Positron emission tomography (PET) seems to be superior to CT (sensitivity, 67–100%). Magnetic resonance imaging (MRI) often offers no advantages when compared with CT, and has higher

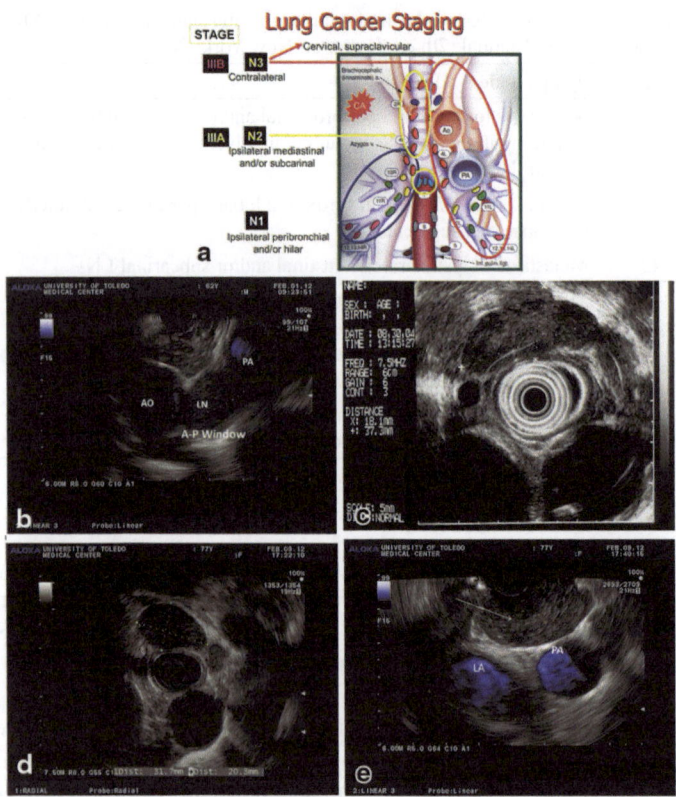

Fig. 4.2. Mediastinal lymph node stations. Diagram of TNM of nonsmall-cell *lung cancer staging* (**a**). Linear EUS showing the aorto-pulmonary window lymph node (**b**), subcarinal lymph node in a case of lung adenocarcinoma (**c**), and *subcarinal* lymph node in a case of lung small cell carcinoma (**d**). Doppler examination is useful to distinguish lymph node from vascular structures (**e**, AP window lymph node linear EUS).

costs. These imaging modalities usually do not procure tissue for diagnosis.

EUS and endoscopic ultrasound fine needle aspiration (EUS-FNA) have a sensitivity of 84–94 % in the evaluation of mediastinal LNs in approachable compartments, and confirm metastatic disease in up to 25 % of patients who show no evidence of mediastinal disease on CT scan (lesions < 1 cm). Similar statistical values, although with lower sensitivity and accuracy, are reported for EUS-FNA in restaging of NSCLC after induction chemotherapy, and are superior to CT or re-mediastinoscopy, which can be technically difficult to perform. The results of EUS-FNA change the management in ~ 80 % of the patients, avoiding thoracotomy/thoracoscopy in up to 49 % and mediastinoscopy in 68 % of cases. EUS-FNA is particularly useful in decreasing the morbidity of image-guided transthoracic FNA and has the potential to prevent unnecessary surgery in patients with mediastinal disease and negative CT scan results.

EUS-FNA reduces NSCLC staging costs by up to 40 % per patient because of the decrease in surgical procedures, namely, mediastinoscopy (~ $ 8000) or exploratory thoracotomy (~ $ 26,000). It is also important that EUS-FNA has 93 % sensitivity vs. 73 % sensitivity of surgical procedures, added to the fact that EUS-FNA can be performed in an ambulatory setting and has lower morbidity (Fig. 4.3).

In summary, EUS-FNA has a high diagnostic yield and accuracy, detects occult metastases, often prevents unnecessary surgery, is cost-effective, and has fewer complications. Thus, initial evaluation with EUS-FNA is recommended instead of mediastinoscopy with biopsy, transbronchial FNA, CT-guided FNA, and PET. According to the European Society of Thoracic Surgery guidelines, mediastinoscopy remains the gold standard for *superior* mediastinal LNs in primary staging of NSCLC; EUS-FNA, EBUS-FNA, and transbronchial FNA are preferred modalities for primary staging of LNs in other locations. Aspiration cytology or surgical modalities may be used for restaging; if negative cytology results, a surgical approach may be indicated, depending on the clinical setting.

We should emphasize that EUS-FNA and EBUS-FNA are complementary in sampling almost all mediastinal compartments and may replace more invasive methods for diagnosing and staging NSCLC. EUS and EUS-FNA have access to paratracheal lymph nodes and lesions located in the posterior and inferior mediastinum. EBUS and EBUS-FNA have access to pretracheal masses and those adjacent to main bronchi particularly in the right side. Sensitivity, specificity, and diagnostic accuracy approach 100 % when both modalities are used.

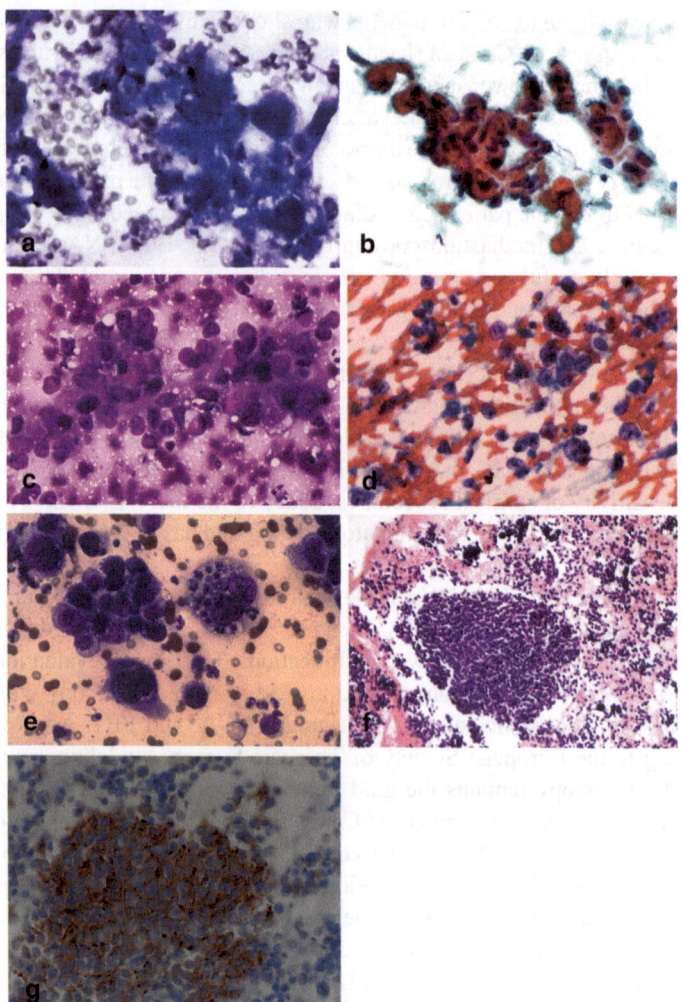

FIG. 4.3. EUS-FNA cytology of lung carcinomas. Examples of metastatic squamous cell carcinoma (**a, b**), adenocarcinoma (**c, d**), large cell undifferentiated carcinoma with giant cell features (**e**), and small cell carcinoma metastatic to mediastinal lymph nodes (**f, g**). (**a, c, e, f** DiffQuik stain, high magnification; **b, d** Papanicolaou stain, high magnification; **g** synaptophysin immunostain, high magnification).

Molecular Markers and Targeted Therapy in Lung Cancer

EUS-FNA is effective in collecting sufficient cytologic material from primary NSCLC or metastatic deposits for performing immunostains (e.g., TTF-1, Napsin A, CEA, and cytokeratin 7 stains for adenocarcinoma) and molecular tests looking for activating mutations of the epidermal growth factor receptor (*EGFR*) gene and rearrangements of anaplastic lymphoma kinase (*ALK*) gene to support the diagnosis of lung adenocarcinoma. EGFR presence is correlated with the response of these tumors to the therapy with tyrosine kinase inhibitors (TKIs) such as gefitinib and erlotinib; ALK presence correlates with response to crizotinib. On the other hand, immunohistochemistry for p63 and/or cytokeratins 5/6 is among the best predictors for diagnosis of squamous cell carcinoma. Severe hemoptysis has been reported in patients with squamous cell carcinoma but not with adenocarcinomas, treated with bevacizumab with or without sorafenib mainly targeted against the vascular endothelial growth factor receptor (VEGFR). Thus, subtyping NSCLC is of paramount importance due to the evidence that cytotoxic chemotherapeutic agents are effective in different forms of NSCLC. However, caution should be taken in evaluating the immunohistochemistry results to make a definitive diagnosis of a lung squamous tumor or an adenocarcinoma in small tissue biopsies or FNA specimens.

Esophageal Cancer

EUS, first introduced in the 1980s is the modality of choice for the evaluation of patients with esophageal carcinoma. EUS is able to evaluate the component layers of the esophageal wall and its adjacent structures and is the most accurate modality for the locoregional (T and N) staging of esophageal cancer.

Most patients with esophageal cancer, in particular adenocarcinoma, present with advanced disease, and the optimal management utilizes stage-dependent algorithms based on both the depth of penetration into the esophageal wall (Fig. 4.4) and the nodal status. Thus, an accurate evaluation is of extreme importance.

Esophageal Cancer Staging

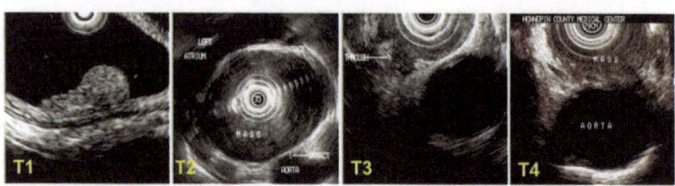

FIG. 4.4. Composite figures showing the ultrasound features of the T-staging of esophageal cancer.

Conventional endoscopic forceps biopsy establishes the primary diagnosis of esophageal cancer. Regional LN metastasis depends on the location of the primary tumor. Cervical or celiac LN metastasis of amid, upper, and lower thoracic esophagus tumor is considered a distant metastasis or M1, as seen in Table 4.3. The tumor is then generally considered unresectable and neoadjuvant chemotherapy or palliative treatment is recommended avoiding unnecessary surgery. Similarly, endomucosal resection is the treatment for patients with T1 (Fig. 4.4) N0 cancers avoiding unnecessary mutilating surgery. Thus, lymph node evaluation is paramount to decide therapy. It must be noted, however, that the clinical importance of celiac lymph node involvement continues to be debated.

Helical CT is most valuable at detecting distant visceral metastatic disease, but is insensitive for detecting the extent of wall involvement (sensitivity 40–60%) or LN metastases measuring < 1 cm. The accuracy of EUS in predicting positive nodal metastasis in esophageal cancer ranges from 70 to 80%. The lymph node sonographic findings by EUS described in Table 4.1 acquire a higher positive predictive value in the presence of T3/4 (see Table 4.3) disease, if > 5 LNs are identified, and celiac region LNs are involved.

The addition of lymph node EUS-FNA increases the sensitivity to 90–100%. EUS-FNA is more sensitive, specific, and accurate than CT and EUS alone for staging of regional and distant LNs and is able to sample LNs ≤ 1 cm (Fig. 4.5). PET scanning can also be

TABLE 4.3. Abbreviated T, N, and M esophageal cancer staging (Fig 4.4). (AJCC Cancer Staging Manual. 7th ed. Springer. New York, 2010).

T (tumor)	
Tis	Carcinoma in situ
T1	Tumor invades lamina propria, muscularis mucosa, or submucosa
T2	Tumor invades muscularis propria
T3	Tumor invades the adventitia
T4	Tumor invades adjacent structures
N (metastasis to regional lymph nodes)	
N1	1–2 LNs
N2	3–6 LNs
N3	≥7 LNs
	Cervical esophagus: upper and lower cervical, scalene, internal jugular, supraclavicular, periesophageal LNs
	UT, MT, and LT esophagus: periesophageal, subcarinal LNs
	Gastroesophageal junction (GEJ) and proximal 5 cm of stomach: lower esophageal, diaphragmatic, pericardial, left gastric, celiac LNs
M (distant metastasis)	
M1	Metastasis to distant organ(s) or to nonregional LNs

UT upper thoracic, *MT* mid thoracic, *LT* lower thoracic, *LN* lymph node

useful for detecting distant and locoregional disease; however, it cannot obtain a tissue diagnosis.

Current optimal staging strategies for esophageal cancer combine EUS-FNA with either CT or PET scans. The combination of CT and EUS-FNA is more cost-effective than PET and EUS-FNA; however, the latter is slightly more effective for detecting celiac node involvement. The accuracy of EUS-FNA in the detection of malignant celiac LNs is almost 100%. By comparison of the clinical outcome of patients before and after the introduction of EUS-FNA, it has been shown that there is a positive impact on patients with esophageal cancer supporting its routine use in staging of this malignancy (Fig. 4.6).

Therapeutic decisions emerge from EUS-FNA nodal status in patients with esophageal cancer. As previously mentioned, patients

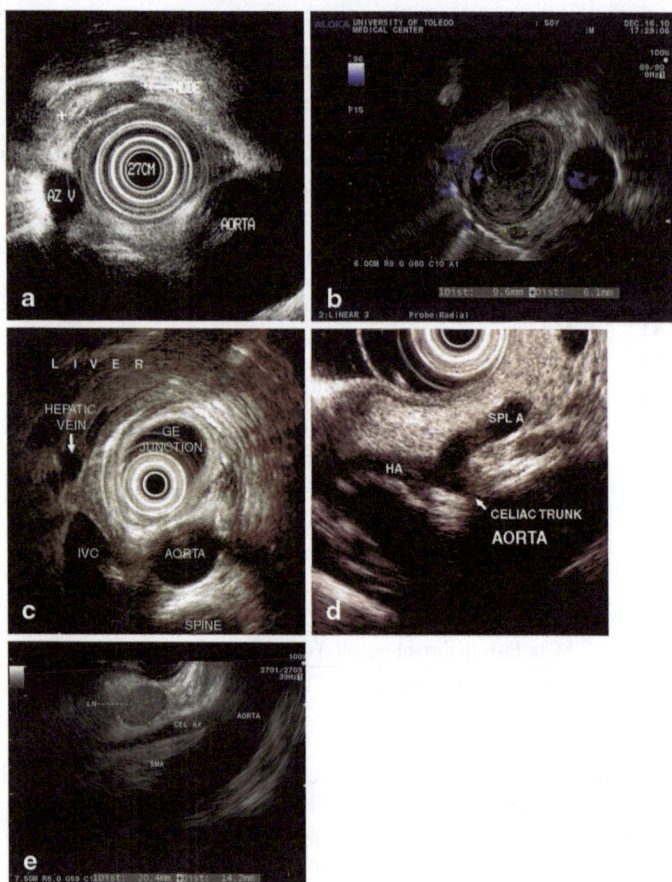

FIG. 4.5. Ultrasound evaluation of the esophagus and regional lymph nodes at 27 cm (**a, b** radial EUS), the GE junction (**c** radial EUS), and posterior gastric to evaluate celiac nodes (**d, e** linear EUS).

with T1 N0 disease will benefit from endomucosal resection. Patients with tumor stage ≥T2 regardless of nodal status may receive neoadjuvant chemotherapy based on the tumor size seen by EUS. EUS-FNA positive lymph nodes help to determine the extent of disease and area for radiation therapy in patients with unresectable tumors.

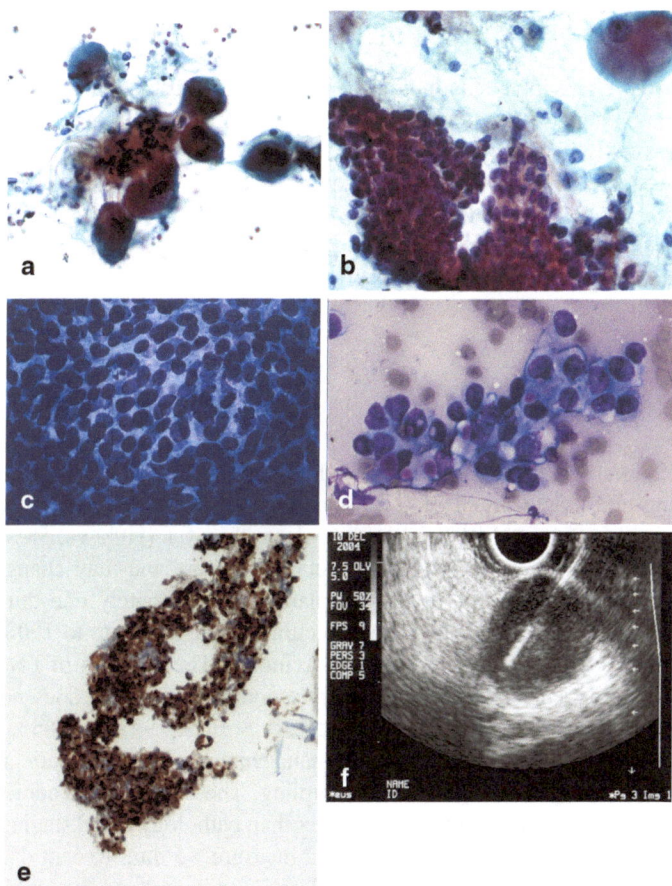

Fɪɢ. 4.6. Cytologic findings of the celiac plexus include fibrous stroma and numerous ganglion cells that may be confused with metastatic malignancy (**a**); a prominent celiac plexus may be mistaken for a lymph node on ultrasound exam. Metastatic adenocarcinoma to celiac lymph node; note one ganglion cell in the *right upper corner* (**b**). Metastatic squamous cell carcinoma of esophagus to a regional lymph node (**c**). Metastatic carcinoma of esophagus with rhabdoid phenotype; note the paranuclear dense cytoplasmic aggregates of intermediate filaments (**d**), that stain positive for vimentin (**e**). EUS-FNA of a sonographically suspicious regional lymph node; the entire needle length is visualized (**f**). (**a**, **b**, Papanicolaou stain, high magnification; **c**, **d**, DiffQuik stain, high magnification; **d**, Immunoperoxidase stain for vimentin in cell block, intermediate magnification).

Gastric Cancer

From endoscopic standpoint, the staging of gastric adenocarcinoma is seen to be analogous to esophageal cancer. Depth of local invasion is accurately assessed and the same sonographic criteria are used to identify lymph nodes that are likely to contain metastatic disease. Likewise, EUS-FNA is accurate 95 % of the time when used for the detection of primary gastric malignancy and nodal metastasis.

Rectal Cancer

Endorectal ultrasound (ERUS) and FNA are important for the staging and management of rectal carcinoma, and for detecting disease recurrence. ERUS is more accurate than CT (90 % vs. 58 %) for determining the T-stage of rectal carcinoma and may change the surgeon's original treatment plan in approximately one third of cases (Fig. 4.7). ERUS-FNA accurately diagnoses up to 100 % of patients with recurrent rectal carcinoma. The addition of FNA shows a trend toward more accurate nodal staging, but does not significantly improve the yield of ERUS alone (92 % vs. 85 %). However, FNA may change the management of 19 % of patients who undergo nonregional LN sampling. The diagnostic accuracy of ERUS nodal staging may be lower than pathology nodal staging, particularly when the LNs involved measure <5 mm. Recent data suggests that MRI may provide a less invasive method for highly accurate T and N classification; however, this does not allow FNA sampling if felt to be clinically necessary.

Anal Cancer

The advantage of endoanal ultrasound (EAUS) in staging of cancer of the anal canal is in the precise assessment of the depth of infiltration and of tumor spread into adjacent tissue, thus facilitating the

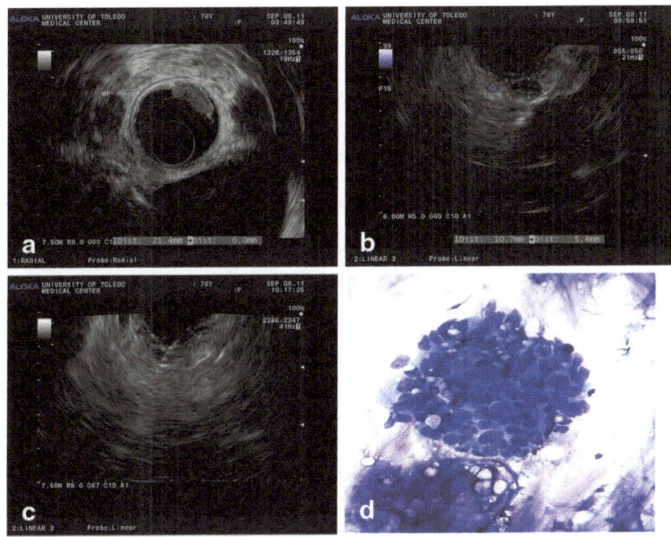

FIG. 4.7. Early rectal adenocarcinoma with small perirectal metastatic lymph node. Radial ERUS shows a 21.4 mm hypoechoic heterogeneous mass with irregular margins particularly in the luminal surface, invading the submucosa and sparing the muscularis propria (MM; **a**). Linear ERUS shows a 10.7×5.4 mm hypoechoic heterogeneous perirectal lymph node with ill-defined and irregular margins (**b**). ERUS-FNA showing the entire needle length and the needle tip within the lymph node (**c**, linear ERUS). Cytology of mucin producing adenocarcinoma (**d**, Romanowsky stain, intermediate magnification).

choice of treatment decisions. The addition of EAUS-FNA for the sampling of suspicious areas may facilitate follow-up examination after the initial treatment.

Further Reading

AJCC. Cancer staging manual 7th ed. New York. Springer; 2010.

Bardales RH, Stelow EB, et al. Review of endoscopic ultrasound-guided fine-needle aspiration cytology. Diagn Cytopathol. 2006;34(2):140–75.

De Angelis C, Pellicano R, et al. Endoscopic ultrasound in the 2013 pre-operative evaluation of gastric cancer. Minerva Gastroenterol Dietol. 2013;59(1):1–12.

Hawes RH. The evolution of endoscopic ultrasound: improved imaging, higher accuracy for fine needle aspiration and the reality of endoscopic ultrasound-guided interventions. Curr Opin Gastroenterol. 2010;26(5):436–44.

Hassan H, Vilmann P, et al. Impact of EUS-guided FNA on management of gastric carcinoma. Gastrointest Endosc. 2010;71(3):500–4.

Hernandez LV, Bhutani MS. Emerging applications of endoscopic ultrasound in gastrointestinal cancers. Gastrointest Cancer Res. 2008;2(4):198–202.

Konge L, Vilmann P, et al. Reliable and valid assessment of competence in endoscopic ultrasonography and fine-needle aspiration for mediastinal staging of non-small cell lung cancer. Endoscopy. 2012;44(10):928–33.

Kundu U, Weston B, Lee J, Hofstetter W, Krishnamurthy S. Evolving role of endoscopic ultrasonography—guided fine-needle aspiration in tumor staging and treatment of patients with carcinomas of the upper gastrointestinal tract. J Am Soc Cytopathol. 2014;3:29–36.

Maleki Z, Erozan Y, et al. Endorectal ultrasound-guided fine-needle aspiration: a useful diagnostic tool for perirectal and intraluminal lesions. Acta Cytol. 2013;57(1):9–18.

Matthes K, Bounds BC, et al. EUS staging of upper GI malignancies: results of a prospective randomized trial. Gastrointest Endosc. 2006;64(4):496–502.

Raptakis T, Boura P, et al. Endoscopic and endobronchial ultrasound-guided needle aspiration in the mediastinal staging of non-small cell lung cancer. Anticancer Res. 2013;33(6):2369–76.

Stelow EB, Lai R, et al. Endoscopic ultrasound-guided fine-needle aspiration of lymph nodes: the Hennepin county medical center experience. Diagn Cytopathol. 2004;30(5):301–6.

Chapter 5
EUS and EUS-FNA of Intramural Masses of the Esophagus, Stomach, and Proximal Intestinal Tract

Ricardo H. Bardales and Shawn Mallery

Endoscopic ultrasound-guided aspiration cytology (EUS-FNA) of intramural lesions of the gastrointestinal (GI) tract is challenging. The first part of this chapter reviews the sonographic anatomy of the GI wall, the most common origin of intramural lesions within the GI wall as seen by ultrasound, and the most common topographic location along the GI tract. This is followed by an extensive description of the cytology of intramural lesions following a pattern-based approach, i.e., spindle, epithelioid, cystic. Histopathology, immunoprofile, molecular profile, and ultrasound features of intramural lesions are also described in addition to the cytologic findings. The last part of the chapter covers EUS-FNA of thick gastric folds. Numerous photomicrographs and pertinent ultrasound pictures complement the text.

R. H. Bardales (✉)
Outpatient Pathology Associates, Pathology and Cytopathology, 7750 College Town Drive Suite 102, Sacramento, CA 95826, USA
e-mail: rhbardales@aol.com

S. Mallery
Division of Gastroenterology, Hepatology and Nutrition, Department of Internal Medicine, University of Minnesota, MMC 36, 420 Delaware St. SE, Minneapolis, MN 55455, USA
e-mail: malle004@umn.edu

R. H. Bardales (ed.), *Cytology of the Mediastinum and Gut Via Endoscopic Ultrasound-Guided Aspiration,* Essentials in Cytopathology 25, DOI 10.1007/978-3-319-12796-5_5,
© Springer International Publishing Switzerland 2015

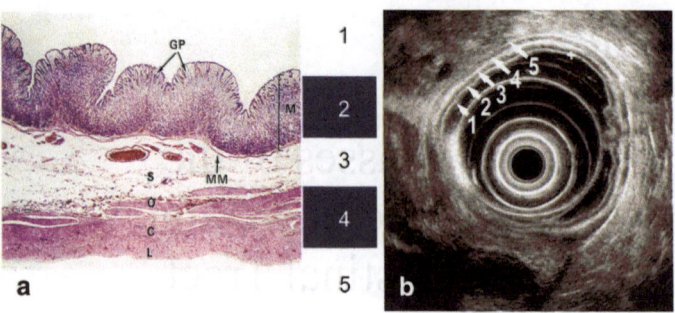

Fɪɢ. 5.1.   Histologic and ultrasound correlation of the GI wall concentric layers. *1.* Mucosa/interface (*clear line*); *2.* Deep mucosa (lamina propria, muscularis mucosa) (*dark line*); *3.* Submucosa (*clear line*); *4.*Muscularis propria (*dark line*); *5.* Serosa/adventitia (*clear line*).

The histologic layers of the normal esophagus and GI tract are the mucosa, muscularis mucosa, submucosa, muscularis propria, and adventitia (in the esophagus) or serosa (in the GI tract). When evaluated at standard endoscopic ultrasound (EUS) frequency of 7.5 MHz, the gut has five alternating, concentric rings (by radial EUS) or parallel layers (by linear EUS): layer 1 (bright, surface interface, epithelium and superficial mucosa), layer 2 (dark, deep mucosa and muscularis mucosa), layer 3 (bright, submucosa), layer 4 (dark, muscularis propria), and layer 5 (bright, adventitia or serosa), which are the result of tissue detail and boundary reflections during ultrasound imaging (Fig. 5.1). High resolution EUS with a 20 MHz miniprobe shows a nine-layer image.

The cytopathologist must be familiar with the EUS anatomy of the GI wall, because some intramural masses may be related to certain layers, favoring one diagnosis over the other, i.e., a gastrointestinal stromal tumor (GIST) generally originates in layer 4 (muscularis propria) (Fig. 5.2). Also important is the echogenicity of the lesion, i.e., hypoechoic (the most common pattern), anechoic, or hyperechoic, which conveys a distinct differential diagnosis (Fig. 5.3). Not less important is the topographic location of the lesion in the GI tract, as seen in Table 5.1.

Combining these characteristics (layer of origin/wall location, GI tract location, and ultrasound pattern) narrows the differential

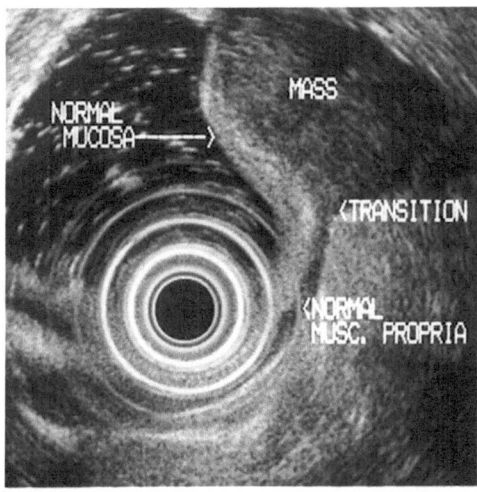

FIG. 5.2.   GIST arising from layer 4 (muscularis propria) of the stomach.

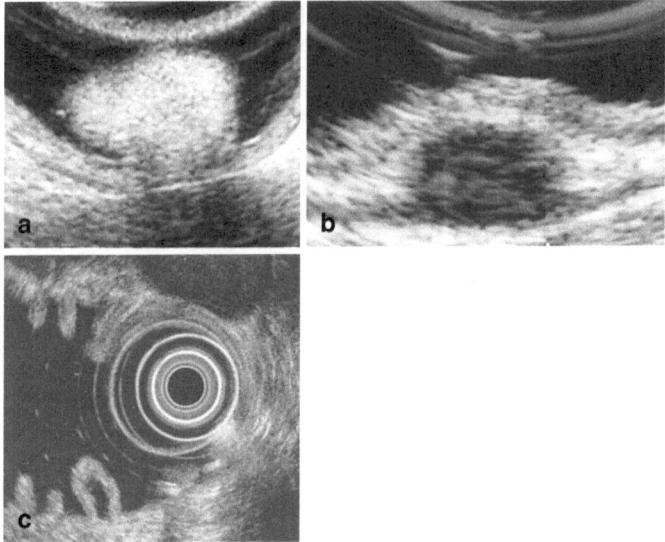

FIG. 5.3.   Echogenicity by EUS: hyperechoic (**a**), hypoechoic (**b**), and anechoic (**c**).

TABLE 5.1.   Where in the gut is the lesion?

Lesion	Most common location(s)
GIST	Stomach, small bowel
Smooth muscle neoplasms	Esophagus, stomach
Signet ring cell carcinoma (diffuse)	Stomach, esophagus
Eosinophilic gastroenteritis	Small bowel, stomach
Congenital cysts	Esophagus, stomach
Heterotopic pancreas	Duodenum, stomach
Granular cell tumor and schwannoma	Esophagus, stomach
Endocrine cell tumor	Rectum, stomach, small bowel
Glomus tumor	Stomach
Brunner's gland heterotopias	Stomach
Brunner's gland hamartoma	Duodenum
Lymphoma	Stomach, small bowel

diagnosis of intramural lesions of the GI tract, as seen in Table 5.2. On note, EUS alone is 30 and 67 % accurate to predict neoplastic and nonneoplastic small (<2 cm) intramural (layers 2 and 3) lesions, respectively, and due to this poor accuracy, these lesions are treated by endomucosal resection with subsequent histopathologic diagnosis. However, depending on the location and size of lesions and operator skill, these lesions may be evaluated by EUS-FNA, avoiding unnecessary resection for a benign lesion such as pancreas rest. Larger intramural lesions (>2 cm) should be sampled by EUS-FNA and the rate of nondiagnostic samples is inverse to mass size (68 % in <2 cm, 13 % in 2–5 cm, and 6 % in >5 cm).

We encourage the pathologist to be aware of the EUS characteristics, relationship to the wall layer, and location of the lesion at time of evaluation to narrow the differential diagnosis.

Intramural Lesions of the Esophagus and Upper GI Tract: A Pattern-Based Diagnosis

EUS is used for diagnosing a variety of GI lesions that cannot be reliably visualized by CT or MRI. The cost-effectiveness of EUS is maximized when EUS-FNA is used to characterize GI intramural

TABLE 5.2.   Where in the GI wall is the lesion?

EUS Layer	Lesions and differential diagnosis
Layer 2 (lamina propria, muscularis mucosa)	Leiomyoma from the muscularis mucosa, neuroendocrine tumor, possibly GIST
	These lesions are rare and almost always hypoechoic
	Due to the superficial nature, these lesions may be accessible to endoscopic mucosal resection or repeated "tunnel" forceps biopsy
Layer 3 (submucosa)	If lesion is hypoechoic: neuroendocrine tumor, pancreas rest, granular cell tumor, schwannoma. Cysts are anechoic; may be hypoechoic
	If lesion is hyperechoic: lipoma, lymphoma, Brunner's gland adenoma, fibroma, and some metastasis
Layer 4 (muscularis propria)	If lesion is hypoechoic: GIST, schwannoma, smooth muscle tumor, metastasis; others are rare
	Hyperechoic lesions such as lipoma are rare in Layer 4

lesions and guide the most appropriate therapy. EUS-FNA is the preferred modality for evaluating and providing an accurate diagnosis, particularly in patients for whom a previous endoscopic forceps biopsy was unsuccessful in establishing a diagnosis. The sensitivity, specificity, and diagnostic accuracy of EUS-FNA in diagnosing such lesions are 89, 88, and 89%, respectively. In contrast, endoscopic forceps biopsy gives a definitive tissue diagnosis in 60% of such cases. Sampling or interpretative errors can result in both false-negative (i.e., gastric lymphoma and GIST) and false-positive (i.e., endometriosis, duodenal diverticulum with muscle hyperplasia, and ectopic pancreas) diagnoses.

In our practice, the initial approach to intramural lesions is with a 25-gauge needle. When EUS is consistent with a mesenchymal neoplasm and rapid interpretation supports such an impression, it is our practice to have the lesion sampled with a 19-gauge needle to obtain material for cell block or to attempt core biopsy (Fig 5.4).

Cytomorphologically, the intramural masses of the esophageal and GI tract can be classified into spindle- and epithelioid-cell

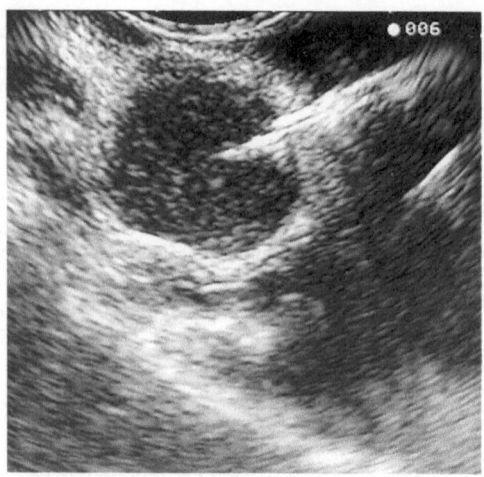

FIG. 5.4.   The initial approach of a mural lesion of the GI tract is with a 25-gauge needle. If material is limited or no material is obtained, then proceed with a 19-gauge needle to obtain not only small tissue fragments for immediate interpretation but also material for a cell block and perform special studies including immunohistochemistry or even molecular tests.

patterns. The latter pattern can be subdivided into large- and small-cell patterns. We will describe the main entities to be considered in the differential diagnosis of these cytologic patterns.

The Spindle-Cell Pattern

GIST, the most common intramural tumor is the prototype of this pattern. The final diagnosis and differentiation from other spindle-cell tumors are essentially based on immunohistochemical analysis applied to cell blocks, as listed in Table 5.3.

TABLE 5.3. GIST: differential diagnosis by immunohistochemistry.

	GIST	SMT	Schwannoma	SFT	IPT	Fibromatosis	Neuroendocrine tumors
CD117[b]	+ memb (95%)	–	–	–	–	– or variable cytoplasmic + (Ab-dependent)	– in low-grade + focal in high-grade
DOG-1[b]	+[a]	–	–	–	–	–	–
CD34	+ diffuse (70%)	+ (10%)	Rarely focal	+	–	Variable focal	–
Desmin	+ focal (20%)	+ strong	–	–	–	Variable focal	–
SMA	+ focal variable	+ strong	–	–	Variable	Variable focal	–
S-100 protein	+ (5%)	–	+			–	
β-catenin[a]	–					+ nuclear	
ALK[a]					+ (60%)		+[a]
Synaptophysin & chromogranin[a]							

GIST gastrointestinal stromal tumor, *SMT* smooth-muscle tumor, *SFT* solitary fibrous tumor, *IPT* inflammatory pseudotumor, *SMA* smooth-muscle actin, *ALK* anaplastic lymphoma kinase, *Ab* antibody, + positive, *memb* membranous, – negative
[a] Markers used in special circumstances
[b] Used when suspect CD117(–) GIST

Gastrointestinal Stromal Tumor (GIST)

GIST is the most common primary nonepithelial neoplasm of the gut. It has a phenotype similar to that of the interstitial cells of Cajal (ICCs), and occurs predominantly in males with a median age of 60 years. However, it can occur in children, with a predilection for girls. The stomach is the most common organ of origin (60–70%) (Fig. 5.5a) followed by the small bowel (20–30%), esophagus, colon, rectum, mesentery, and omentum (all <10%). In general, GISTs have an unpredictable behavior; however, GISTs arising in the stomach are less likely to be malignant than those arising in the small bowel, peritoneum, or omentum. Prognosis is based on three parameters: size, tumor location, and proliferation (mitotic) index. GIST can occur in patients with type I neurofibromatosis, pulmonary chordomas, and/or extraadrenal paragangliomas. When possible, complete surgical resection of the tumor is the treatment of choice for localized GIST; however, for inoperable or metastatic tumors, imatinib mesylate (Gleevec®), a c-kit tyrosine kinase receptor inhibitor approved by the FDA in February 2002, is the drug of choice. Sunitinib malate was approved by the FDA in February 2006 for the treatment of patients with recurrent GIST that developed secondary resistance to, or cannot tolerate Gleevec®. The recently FDA-approved (February 2013) regorafenib (Stivarga®), an oral multikinase inhibitor that targets angiogenic, stromal, and oncogenic tyrosine kinase receptors may be used in patients with advanced GIST that cannot be removed and do not respond to imatinib and sunitinib.

Histopathology Most GISTs (approximately 70%) have a spindle-cell pattern (Fig. 5.5b). Tumors are composed of interlacing fascicles or whorls of bland-appearing spindle cells with elongated nuclei showing blunt tips, and slightly eosinophilic cytoplasm. The stroma may be sclerosed, hyalinized, or calcified. Tumor cellularity is variable and pleomorphism is uncommon, but is associated with malignant potential. Prognostic factors for aggressive behavior include size, mitotic index (number of mitoses per 50 high-powered fields (HPF)), mucosal invasion and/or ulceration, and cystic or

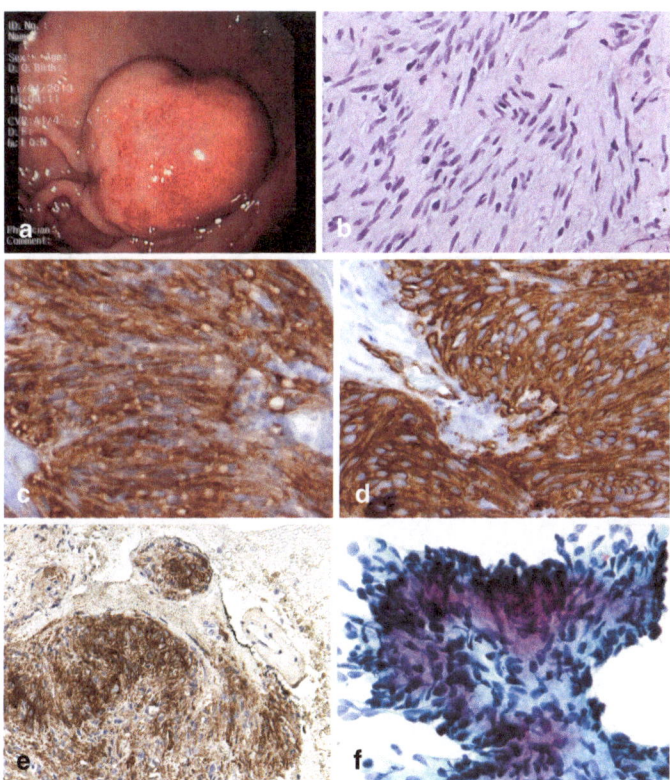

Fɪɢ. 5.5.   Gastrointestinal stromal tumor, spindle-cell pattern. Endo-scopic view of a submucosal mass in the gastric body (**a**). Tissue section shows fascicles of bland-appearing spindle cells with blunt ends arranged in a palisade fashion mimicking a neurogenic origin (**b**). Immunostains are posi-tive for CD117 (**c**), CD34 (**d**), and DOG1 (**e**). Smears show interlacing fas-cicles of uniform spindle cells with slight cell dissociation in the periphery of the cell aggregates (**f**); nuclear palisading is evident (**g**). Fragments of normal submucosa (**h**) and smooth muscle (**i**) are less cellular and exhibit less cell dis-sociation. EUS shows a hypoechoic and heterogeneous intramural mass with smooth and well-defined margins (**j**). Ultrasound features suggestive for an aggressive behavior include hyperchoic foci (**k**), irregular tumor margins (**l**), and cystic degeneration (**m**). (**b**, H&E stain intermediate magnification; **c–e** Immunoperoxidase stain intermediate magnification; **f** Papanicolaou stain in-termediate magnification; **g–i** DiffQuik stain intermediate magnification).

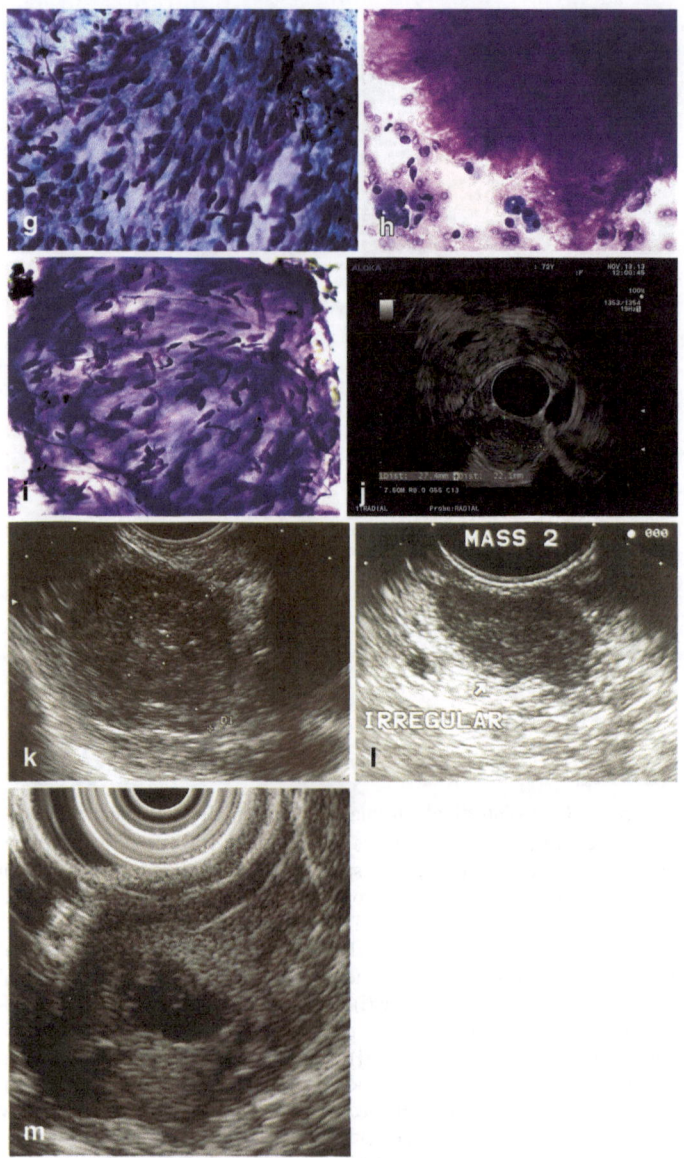

FIG. 5.5.   (continued)

necrotic areas within the tumor, all best assessed in resected specimens. Based on tumor size and mitotic count per 50 HPF, the National Institute of Health proposed a consensus to classify GISTs into very low, low, intermediate, and high risk categories. GISTs of <2 cm and <2 mitotic index have a very low risk of aggressive behavior; GISTs of >5 cm and >5 mitotic index as well as >10 cm or >10 mitotic index regardless of mitotic index or size respectively have a high risk. Proliferation markers such as Ki67 >10% can be more objective than the mitotic index. Ezrin, p16, low apoptosis, high telomerase, and vascular endothelial cell markers have been described as predictors of aggressive behavior. Although most patients with intermediate or lower risk behave in a benign manner, less than 10% of GISTs in such patients will have an unpredicted behavior. Therefore, no lesion can be definitely labeled as benign. For the same reason, all GISTs should be excised, and patients are carefully and regularly followed indefinitely. Special mention goes to colonic GIST which is more common and more aggressive than leiomyosarcoma, and is usually identified late in the course of the disease, underscoring the usefulness of immunohistochemistry in the diagnosis.

Gastrointestinal autonomic nerve tumor (GANT), originally described as plexosarcoma (based on the ultrastructural resemblance to cells of the autonomic nervous system), is a phenotypic variant of GIST. It has the same immunohistologic phenotype (CD117+) and genotype (*c-kit* gene mutation) as does GIST.

Normally, there are CD117+ cells in the omentum, just underneath the mesothelial lining, that may be the origin for extragastrointestinal (E) GISTs. EGISTs are more likely to have epithelioid cell morphology, arise in the omentum and mesentery, behave like small-bowel tumors, and have CD117 expression similar to GISTs. The pattern of *c-kit* and platelet-derived growth factor receptor-α *(PDGFRA)* gene mutations is similar to GIST and plays an important role in tumorigenesis of EGIST. Thus, Gleevec® seems to provide a therapeutic strategy for advanced EGIST. It should be stressed that GISTs should be defined by virtue of any degree of association with the muscularis propria of the gut (no matter how minimal), and not by localization of the bulk of the tumor; keeping this in mind, Agaimy et al. identified that only 1.5% of 200 tumors initially considered to be EGISTs after extensive pathologic exam were found to be truly EGISTs.

Immunoprofile CD117 cytoplasmic and/or membranous positivity is detected in 95% of GISTs (the pattern is usually cytoplasmic with membranous accentuation). CD34 (a hematopoietic stem-cell marker) shows diffuse strong cytoplasmic staining in 70% of cases, with the least positivity in small-bowel tumors; colonic GISTs rarely stain with CD34 (Table 5.3). Staining with other markers is more variable: BCL-2 (80%), smooth-muscle actin (SMA, 40%), S-100 protein (5%). Positive CD117 and CD34 staining in the appropriate clinical context with compatible microscopic features confirms the diagnosis of these tumors (Fig. 5.5c, d). Appropriate positive and negative controls must be run simultaneously. h-caldesmon (an actin-binding cytoskeleton-associated protein) and calponin are positive in 80 and 25% of GISTs, respectively.

Approximately 5% of GISTs have a negative CD117 phenotype. These are histologically and clinically similar to CD117(+) GISTs; however, they are more likely to have epithelioid cell morphology, contain *PDGFRA* oncogenic mutations, and arise in the omentum/peritoneal surface as EGISTs. It has been shown that some CD117(−) GISTs contain Gleevec-sensitive *PDGFRA* or *c-kit* gene mutations and may still benefit from Gleevec® therapy.

New immunomarkers such as CD171 (L1), a cell adhesion molecule, and DOG1 (Fig. 5.5e), a protein of unknown function, are positive in GIST and are expressed independently of *c-kit* or *PDG-FRA* gene mutations; they are useful for the diagnosis of CD117(−) GIST. CD117 and DOG1 each stain >95% of GISTs, and stain all GISTs when both are used together.

Not every CD117(+) tumor is a GIST; i.e., synovial sarcoma, malignant fibrous histiocytoma, dermatofibrosarcoma protuberans, and vascular tumors, among others, may react at least focally with antibodies directed against CD117. Fortunately, most do not occur in the gut. Metastatic spindle-cell melanoma can be distinguished based on clinical and imaging findings as well as on S100 protein positivity. DOG1 is rarely expressed in other mesenchymal tumors.

Molecular Profile Genes encoding for the c-kit receptor and PDG-FRA of the tyrosine kinase subfamily are located in chromosome 4 and are important in the pathogenesis of GIST. KIT (a transmembrane glycoprotein) has a receptor for stem cell factor (SCF), and it has been shown that mice deficient in KIT or SCF fail to develop ICCs, indicating that this axis is critical for the development of these pacemaker cells. Binding of SCF ligand to KIT produces dimerization of KIT, which activates tyrosine kinase, resulting in phosphorylation of substrates and activation of signal transduction cascades. This leads to well-controlled cell functions (proliferation, adhesion, apoptosis, and differentiation) of hematopoietic progenitor cells, melanocytic cells, mast cells, germ cells, and ICCs. KIT glycoprotein is recognized by the CD117 antibody. CD117 is expressed in ICCs and in GISTs, substantiating the hypothesis that GISTs arise from or share a common stem cell with the ICCs and providing a new specific and sensitive marker for the diagnosis of GIST.

Most GISTs express activated KIT oncoproteins, and thus the activation does not depend on binding SCF ligand (in contrast to KIT glycoprotein). KIT oncoproteins in GISTs commonly have oncogenic mutations of the *c-kit* juxtamembrane domain, exon 11, and less commonly exons 9, 13, and 17, which results in a ligand-independent KIT dimerization and activation of the tyrosine kinase, followed by receptor autophosphorylation, activation of intracellular signaling cascades, and ultimately aberrant cell proliferation, apoptosis, chemotaxis, and adhesion. It is interesting to note that various mutations have different responses to Gleevec®, i.e., *c-kit* mutations (exon 11, excellent response; exon 9, intermediate response; exon 17, resistant) and *PDGFRA* mutations (exon 12, sensitive; exon 18, poor response). GISTs exhibit typical activating mutations of *c-kit* and less commonly in the *PDGFRA* protooncogenes; however, 15 % are negative for these two mutations. Pediatric GISTs often have no *c-kit* (exons 9, 11, 13, and 17) or *PDG-FRA* (exons 12, 14, and 18) mutations (wild type). Some wild-type GISTs may show *c-kit* exon 8 mutations and be imatinib-sensitive. Wild-type GISTs may have various oncogenic mutations such as neufibromatosis (*NF*) type I, *RAS*, and *BRAF* V600E (13 % of wild-type cases) genes. Of note, 7% of patients with NF1 develop GISTs, mainly in the small bowel. The recently described succinate dehydrogenase- (SDH) deficient GISTs are always wild-type, show an epithelioid morphology, and often occur in association with the Carney triad.

Lastly, molecular analysis of GISTs, looking for the various mutations, can be done in paraffin-embedded cell-block samples obtained by EUS-FNA. This molecular analysis is a step forward in the diagnosis from a small sample. We should emphasize that since type and dose of tyrosine kinase inhibitors depends on the mutation identified, routine genotyping is strongly recommended for appropriate GIST management.

FNA Findings EUS-FNA cytology smears show variable numbers of spindle cells arranged in fairly cellular and cohesive short fascicles or whorls. The spindle cells are uniform and show indistinct cytoplasmic borders, giving a syncytial aspect to the fragment. Nuclei are elongated, with blunt ends and small inconspicuous nucleoli in a fibrillary background stroma. Variable numbers of single stripped nuclei are usually scattered mostly at the periphery of the cell fragments. The spindle cells are aligned in a Schwannian pattern, with prominent nuclear palisading mimicking schwannoma (Fig. 5.5 f, g). The stromal collagen is minimal. Mitosis, necrosis, and cell pleomorphism may be indicators of aggressive behavior. The cell block usually shows a densely cellular spindle-cell pattern and may show juxtanuclear vacuoles and palisading. Juxtanuclear vacuoles are seen in ~5% of all GISTs, and particularly in gastric tumors. It has been observed that malignant gastric GISTs tend to lose these vacuoles.

GISTs can be misinterpreted as benign fibrous tissue or fragments of smooth muscle of the GI wall that one might encounter in a routine transmural EUS-FNA (Fig. 5.5h, i). Larger cell size and haphazardly arranged cell fascicles are clues in favor of GIST over normal gut wall fragments. When smears and cell blocks are combined, EUS-FNA is accurate in the diagnosis of GIST. The accuracy of EUS and EUS-FNA for the diagnosis of probably malignant GIST is 78 and 91%, respectively. EUS-FNA with Ki-67 immunoshistochemical stain is an accurate, sensitive, and specific method for differentiating potentially aggressive from less aggressive GISTs. In our experience, GISTs, schwannomas, and leiomyomata share a similar cytomorphology, and only cell-block immunostain results help to differentiate one from the other. The differential diagnosis also includes fibromatosis (nuclear catenin +), sclerosing mesenteritis (nuclear catenin −), inflammatory myofibroblastic tumor, and spindle cell-neuroendocrine tumors (synaptophysin + and chromogranin +); the distinction is based mainly on immunohistochemistry (Fig. 5.6a–e, Table 5.3).

EUS Features Lesions are hypoechoic and covered by sonographically and endoscopically normal mucosa (occasionally with small areas of ulceration) (Fig. 5.5j). Generally, a point of attachment is identified between the mass and the muscularis propria (Fig. 5.2); however, this may at times be unapparent. The EUS features that predict an adverse behavior include hyperechoic foci, irregular margins, cystic spaces, and size > 5 cm (Fig. 5.5k–m).

Leiomyoma and Leiomyosarcoma

Although rare elsewhere in the GI tract, leiomyomas are the most common esophageal mesenchymal neoplasms. Leiomyomas are 5 times more common than GISTs in the esophagus and 50 times less common than GISTs in the stomach and small bowel. Gastric and small-bowel smooth-muscle tumors are exceedingly rare (Fig. 5.7a). Most leiomyomas of the GI tract are sporadic but they may occur in association with Alport syndrome (hearing loss and renal disease) and multiple endocrine neoplasia (MEN) type 1 syndrome (pituitary and parathyroid adenomas, and pancreas neuroendocrine tumor). Most, if not all esophageal leiomyomas involve the entire esophageal wall and are clinically indolent intramural tumor masses with no tumor-related mortality. Patients usually seek help for dysphagia. However, leiomyomas are also found incidentally during endoscopic work-up for other causes. Colorectal leiomyomas are occasionally found incidentally as polyps on screening colonoscopy and are more common than colorectal GISTs.

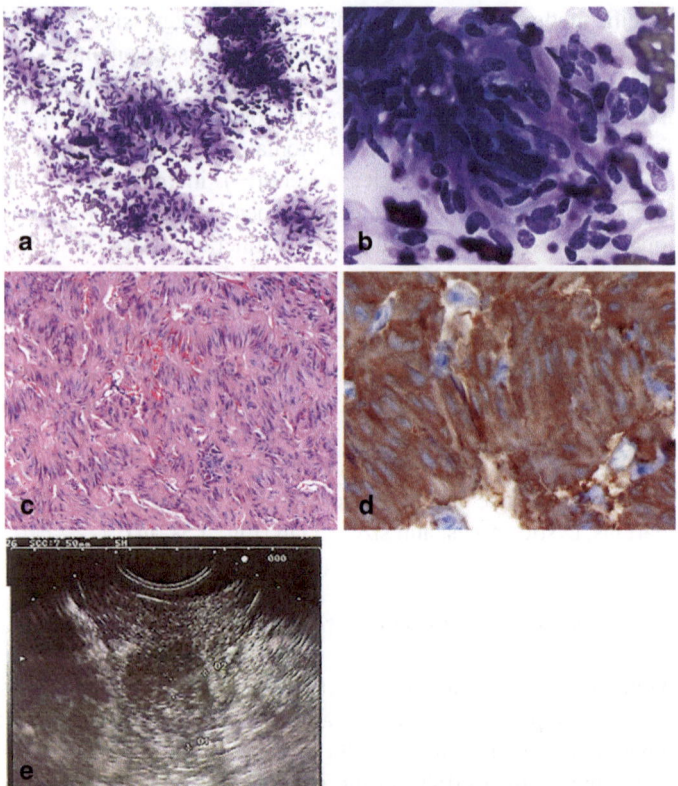

Fig. 5.6.   Spindle-cell neuroendocrine tumor. A trabecular and nested
pattern composed of bland-appearing spindle cells embedded in a dense
and fibrillary stroma (**a**, **b**). Histopathology (**c**) recapitulates the EUS-FNA
pattern, which stains positive for synaptophysin (**d**). Ultrasound features
a hypoechoic heterogeneous solid mass involving the submucosa with no
involvement of the muscularis propria (**e**). (**a**, **b** DiffQuik stain, low- and
high-magnification; **c**, H&E stain, low magnification; **d** Immunoperoxidase stain, high magnification).

Leiomyosarcomas of the GI tract are much less common than
GISTs and can occur anywhere in the tract; however, esophageal
and gastric leiomyosarcomas are exceedingly rare. The incidence

increases in the small bowel and colorectum. Of note, colorectal leiomyosarcomas are ten times less common than colorectal GISTs. Most GI tract leiomyosarcomas follow an aggressive course. Small tumors may have a good prognosis, better than GISTs of the same size and proliferation rate.

Histopathology Leiomyomas show fascicles of spindle cells with eosinophilic cytoplasm and cigar-shaped nuclei that have blunt ends (Fig. 5.7b). Atypia, mitoses, and necrosis are seen in leiomyosarcoma; however, they may have features overlapping with those of leiomyoma. Large size (>5 cm), intratumoral necrosis or hemorrhage, and a mitotic count >5 per HPF are features suggestive of leiomyosarcoma. Colorectal leiomyosarcomas are typically transmural, with both intraluminal and outward-bulging components, and they are more often spindle shaped than epithelioid (rate 9:1). The differential diagnosis includes GIST, spindle-cell carcinoma, and amelanotic melanoma.

Immunoprofile Immunohistochemistry for smooth-muscle markers conclusively defines these lesions and can be performed readily in the cell block. Leiomyomas are positive for desmin and SMA (Fig. 5.7c), and negative for CD117, CD34, and S-100 protein. Leiomyosarcoma shows positive smooth-muscle markers (Fig. 5.7d), but no CD117 (Table 5.3). They are also positive for calponin and h-caldesmon.

FNA Findings Smears show clusters of elongated cells with bland nuclei and rare, if any, mitoses. Cell nuclei are placed in an abundant stroma. DiffQuik stain may show a dense glassy stroma. Papanicolaou stain shows the characteristic eosinophilia in the cytoplasm (Fig. 5.7e, f).

In our experience, except for the low-group cellularity and lack of background stripped nuclei observed in leiomyomata, the cytomorphologic features of leiomyomata observed in DiffQuik-stained smears are similar to those of GISTs. Scattered stripped nuclei with scant fibrillary cytoplasm present in a more cellular, haphazardly arranged fragment are commonly seen in GIST, in

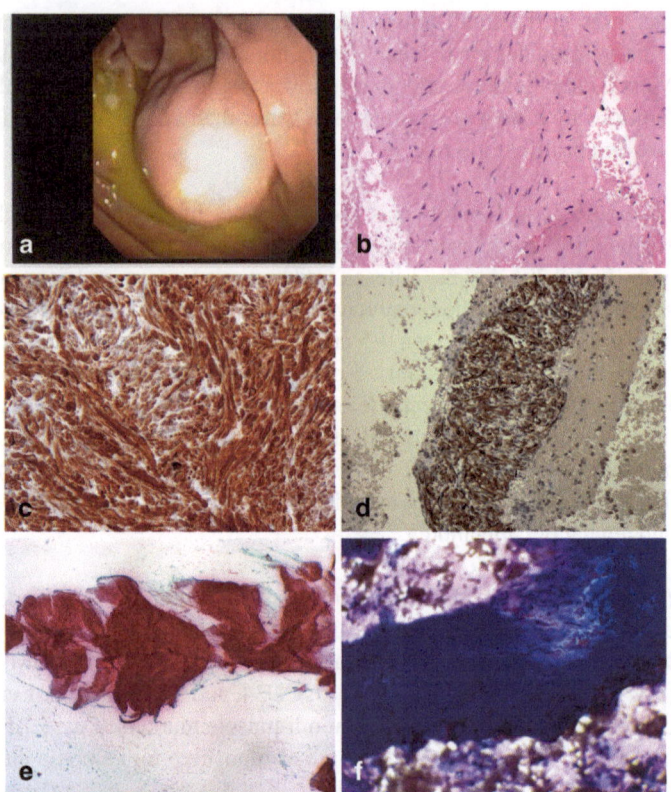

FIG. 5.7. Leiomyoma and leiomyosarcoma. Endoscopic view of a gastric fundus submucosal mass (**a**). Note the eosinophilic glassy stroma
surrounding spindle cells (**b**). Smooth-muscle actin stain is positive in
leiomyoma (**c**) and leiomyosarcoma (**d**). The eosinophilic stroma is best
seen in the Papanicolaou stain (**e**) and the glassy features in the DiffQuik
stain (**f**). Fragments of muscularis propria (**g**) are impossible to distinguish
from those of leiomyoma (**h**). Cellular pleomorphism is present in leiomyosarcoma (**i**). EUS of leiomyoma showing a hypoechoic gastric fundus submucosal mass (31.2 × 29.5 mm) with central anechoic cystic space
(*MP* muscularis propria) (**j**). (**b**, H&E stain intermediate magnification; **c**,
d Immunoperoxidase stain for actin intermediate magnification; **e**, **g** & **i**
Papanicolaou stain low and high magnification; **f**, **h** DiffQuik stain intermediate magnification).

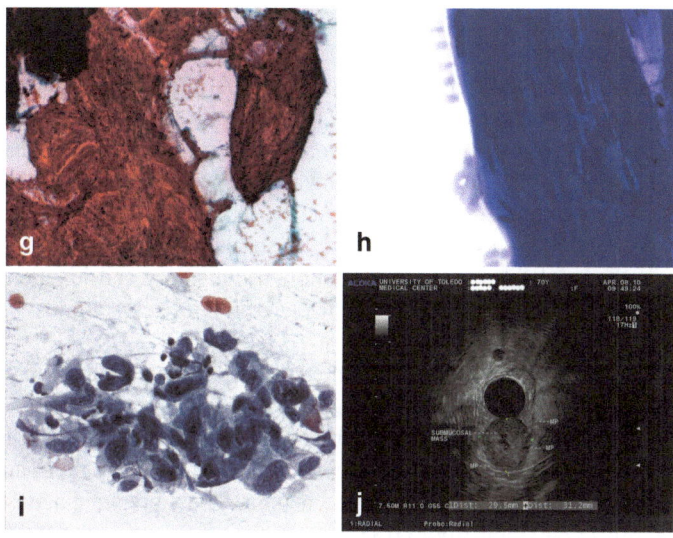

FIG. 5.7.   (continued)

contrast to leiomyoma. The characteristic eosinophilic cytoplasm of leiomyoma is best seen in cell-block slides. Cells may be more ovoid, less crowded, lack schwannoid features, and have greater cell cohesion in leiomyoma. The distinction of leiomyoma from normal smooth muscle from the GI wall is more problematic. They may have similar cytologic features, particularly in marginally sampled leiomyomas; ultrasound correlation assuring that the mass was sampled is necessary for a correct interpretation (Fig. 5.7g, h). Leiomyosarcoma often shows marked cellular pleomorphism (Fig. 5.7i).

EUS Features Tumors may arise from either layer 2 or layer 4. The sonographic features by themselves are indistinguishable from those of GIST. Leiomyomas are hypoechoic, with homogeneous echotexture, oval or round, and have well-defined margins (Fig. 5.7j). Malignant tumors are hypoechoic, have irregular infiltrating margins, fuzzy borders, and may show heterogeneous echotexture that indicates necrosis.

Schwannoma

Although most mesenchymal tumors of the gut are GISTs, other mesenchymal tumors, including nerve sheath tumors, do occur. Like GISTs, schwannomas are more frequent in the stomach than in other GI locations. Colonic schwannomas are sometimes found incidentally on screening colonoscopy. These tumors are not associated with neurofibromatosis. Ultrastructural findings are those of peripheral schwannomas and show rudimentary cell junctions, basal lamina, and intracytoplasmic electron-dense crystalloids.

Histopathology Schwannomas are not encapsulated, show interlacing cell fascicles, are surrounded by a lymphoid cuff with germinal centers, and have intratumoral lymphoid cells. In contrast to GISTs, GI schwannomas do not have a schwannoid pattern and may be mitotically active and be benign. Thus, proper diagnosis and differentiation from GIST is important because of the difference in prognosis and therapy (Fig. 5.8a).

Immunoprofile In our laboratory: a panel of CD117, CD34, S-100 protein, desmin, and SMA is routinely applied to spindle-cell tumors of the GI tract. S-100 protein (+) and CD117(−) applied to cell blocks are confirmatory of schwannoma (Fig. 5.8d). CD34 may be focally positive. In contrast with peripheral schwannomas, calretinin is negative.

Molecular Profile GI schwannomas usually lack *NF2* gene alterations, in contrast to peripheral schwannomas.

FNA Findings Schwannomas show moderately cellular groups that may have haphazardly arranged bland cells within a dense stroma when stained with DiffQuik. Nuclei may be oval, elongated, or round and only occasionally wavy. The stroma is fibrillary when stained with Papanicolaou stain. In contrast to GIST and similar to leiomyoma, stripped nuclei are only occasionally present in the smear background. Rarely, these tumors may be epithelioid. Nuclear palisading and Verrocay bodies, so characteristic of peripheral

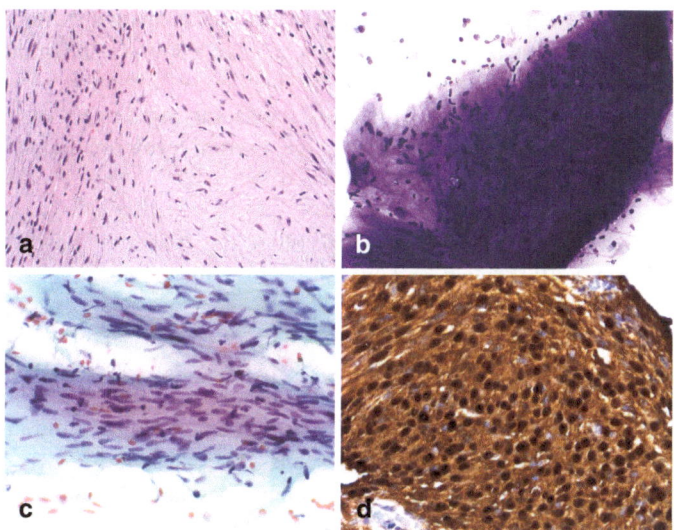

Fig. 5.8.   Schwannoma. Histologic (**a**) and EUS-FNA (**b, c**) findings are indistinguishable from those of spindle-cell GIST. Stain for S-100 protein is required for final characterization (**d**). (**a**, H&E stain intermediate magnification; **b** DiffQuik stain high magnification; **c** Papanicolaou stain high magnification; **d** nuclear stain for S-100 protein, intermediate magnification).

schwannomas, are virtually absent in GI schwannomas (Figs. 5.8b, c). Furthermore, schwannoid features are not uncommonly seen in GISTs (Figs. 5.5g).

EUS Features Similar to GIST, schwannoma arises in the fourth layer (muscularis propria) of the GI wall and is hypoechoic, round to oval, and has well-defined margins and homogeneous echotexture.

Sclerosing Mesenteritis

This entity is an IgG4-related disease, recognized as a systemic syndrome characterized by mass-forming lesions in the pancreas, retroperitoneum, mesentery, lung, head, and neck, with lymphoplasmacytic infiltration and sclerosis. Patients with sclerosing mesenteritis are usually adults who have a solitary abdominal mass involving the mesentery of the small bowel without involvement of the bowel wall. This mass shows varying degrees of inflammation, necrosis, and fibrosis. IgG4 serum levels are high and are helpful in the diagnosis.

Immunoprofile CD117, CD34, and SMA may be focally positive. Desmin, S-100 protein, and nuclear beta-catenin are negative.

Mesenteric Fibromatosis

This tumor, also named intraabdominal desmoid tumor, infiltrates the bowel wall, has interlacing fascicles, and lacks fat necrosis or inflammation. Most mesenteric fibromatoses have mutations in the beta-catenin pathway and have an abnormal nuclear accumulation of beta-catenin protein, which is helpful in the differential diagnosis.

Immunoprofile Mesenteric fibromatosis may show weak focal or diffuse CD117 and focal actin and desmin positivity, in keeping with myofibroblastic differentiation, but is negative for DOG-1, CD34, and S-100 protein (Table 5.3). Both PDGFRs and their ligands are expressed. Nuclear beta-catenin is positive in almost all cases and cyclin D-1 in 65 %.

Inflammatory Pseudotumor (IPT)

This process is also called plasma cell granuloma. Tissue sections show myofibroblastic spindle cells and an intense plasma cell infiltrate admixed with lymphocytes. Patients are in the first two decades of life and have an abdominal mass, fever, leukocytosis, a high sedimentation rate, and anemia.

Immunoprofile CD117, CD34, and desmin are negative. SMA is variably positive (Table 5.3).

Molecular Profile Clonal cytogenetic abnormalities involving the anaplastic lymphoma kinase (*ALK*) gene on chromosome arm 2p have been identified in IPT. Thus, ALK is positive in these tumors and is helpful for the diagnosis.

Inflammatory Fibroid Polyp (IFP)

These lesions are seen in adults with a slight female preponderance; usually affect the gastric antrum and large intestine with predominance of the rectosigmoid, and patients are usually asymptomatic. However, they often have intussusception when IFP affects the small intestine. The size of the lesion is variable and may be large as 12 cm and cause gastric-outlet obstruction, although it usually measures 1–2 cm. These lesions are frequently pedunculated and amenable to endoscopic snare excision.

Histopathology This benign intramural lesion has variable cellularity and vascularity. It is composed of short fascicles of bland-appearing spindle cells, rich vasculature, and inflammatory cells rich in eosinophils. Spindle cells distributed around vessels or "onion skinning" in a myxoid stroma are characteristic; however, this characteristic pattern is present in 50 % of cases. Mitosis and necrosis are absent. Approximately 10 % of patients with gastric IFP have an adenocarcinoma or adenoma in the same area.

Immunoprofile This lesion is CD34- and vimentin-positive. Reactivity with SMA and CD68 may be present. Keratin, CD117, S-100 protein, and EMA are negative.

Molecular Profile IFPs have mutations in the *PDGFR-A* gene exons 12 and 18, raising the possibility of the lesion being neoplastic instead of reactive as was previously considered.

EUS Features Reported EUS features of IFP include an indistinct margin, hypoechoic homogeneous echotexture, and location within the second and/or third layer of the wall, with an intact fourth layer.

Calcifying Fibrous Tumor of the Stomach

Most of these tumors involve the muscularis propria of the stomach (it may occur in the small bowel) with variable submucosal and subserosal extension. It occurs in adults, with no gender predilection. Histologically, bundles of hyalinized collagen predominate, and rare cellular spindle-cell fibroblastic areas are present. Lymphocytes, plasma cells, and aggregates of psammomatous calcifications are also identified. Local resection is the treatment of choice, and the prognosis is excellent, with rare recurrences. These tumors are distinct from other spindle-cell lesions of the stomach and may represent a localized fibrosclerotic inflammatory response.

Immunoprofile CD117, SMA, desmin, S-100 protein, h-caldesmon, and PDGFRA are negative. Focal CD34 + may be seen. In rare cases, ALK may be focally positive.

EUS Features In a case report, EUS showed a focal hypoechoic lesion involving the gastric wall associated with intralesional hyperechoic foci. Marked posterior acoustic shadowing due to calcium deposits precluded examination of the deep margins of the lesion.

Plexiform Fibromyxoma

These tumors are usually located in the gastric antrum and may extend to the perigastric soft tissue. Histologically, the tumors show a plexiform intramural growth with multiple, variably cellular myxoid to collagenous and fibromyxoid micronodules. The tumor cells show mild atypia and mitotic activity < 5/50 HPF. Plexiform fibromyxoma is a distinctive benign gastric antral neoplasm that should be separated from GIST, nerve-sheath tumors, and other fibromyxoid neoplasms.

Immunoprofile SMA is positive. CD10 is variably positive. CD117, DOG1, CD34, desmin, and S-100 protein are all negative.

Malignant Fibrous Histiocytoma (MFH)

Primary or metastatic MFH may involve the stomach, exhibit pleomorphic histologic features, and should be distinguished from a variety of primary and metastatic pleomorphic neoplasms, including high-grade sarcomatous GISTs, pleomorphic leiomyosarcoma, and sarcomatoid carcinoma.

Immunoprofile SMA and PDGFRA are commonly positive and show a myo/fibroblastic phenotype. CD117, CD34, and S-100 protein are negative.

Molecular Profile Primary gastric MFHs reported were wild-type for *KIT* and *PDGFRA*.

The Epithelioid Large-Cell Pattern (Table 5.4)

Epithelioid GIST

Epithelioid GISTs (20 % of GISTs) have also been termed leiomyoblastomas or epithelioid smooth-muscle tumors, which occur more often in the gastric antrum. A mixed spindle and epithelioid histologic pattern is seen in 10 % of GISTs. EGISTs and GISTs that occur in children are often epithelioid and commonly affect the stomach. These patients may harbor a succinate dehydrogenase-(SDH) deficient GIST, which is a unique class of GIST. Malignant GISTs also are often epithelioid.

Histopathology Cells with clear, signet ring, oxyphilic, and plasmacytoid features are arranged in nests or cohesive sheets. Cytoplasmic vacuoles may be prominent, pushing the nuclei to the periphery. Nuclei may be round, oval, or pleomorphic, and the nucleoli may range from inconspicuous to prominent and eosinophilic. Thus, the histologic pattern ranges from epithelioid to overly sarcomatous. Mitotic activity is variable and, as in spindle-cell GIST, is related to tumor behavior. Epithelioid GISTs may be confused with

TABLE 5.4. Epithelioid large-cell pattern: cytology and immunohisto-chemistry.

	GIST	Lymphoma	Carcinoma	GCT	Melanoma
Cytology	Ample eosinophilic cytoplasm. Spindle-cell component is variable	Dissociated cells. Variable cytoplasm. Round nuclei. Variable nucleoli	Aggregates and single, often pleomorphic cells	Granular eosinophilic cytoplasm	Variable cell pleomorphism. Intranuclear inclusions
CD117	+	−	−	−	+
DOG-1	+	−	−	−	−
CD34	+	−	−	−	−
CD45	−	+	−	−	−
Keratin	−	−	+	−	−
S-100 protein	−	−	−	+	+
HMB45	−	−	−	−	+

GIST gastrointestinal stromal tumor, GCT granular cell tumor, + positive, − negative

carcinomas, neuroendocrine tumors, melanomas, and other epithelioid mesenchymal neoplasms (Fig. 5.9a).

Immunoprofile DOG1 and CD171 are positive. Most tumors are CD117 and CD34 positive (Fig. 5.9b). However, occasionally reactivity with CD117 is weak or even negative, and CD34 may also be negative. Immunoreactivity with CD117 and CD34 may be lost after imatinib therapy. In mixed spindle epithelioid GISTs (~10%), staining of the spindle-cell component with CD117 is commonly stronger than the epithelioid component; a sole cytoplasmic paranuclear dotlike- or mixed with diffuse cytoplasmic staining is seen in approximately 40% of cases. SDH-deficient GIST immunostains are positive for CD117 and DOG1 and negative for SDH-B.

Molecular Profile Epithelioid GISTs often have mutations in the *PDGFRA* gene and may have a good prognosis. Activating mutations of the *c-KIT* gene are less common than in spindle-cell GISTs.

SDH-deficient GISTs are wild type for c-*KIT* and *PDGFRA*, occur in the stomach, have an epithelioid histomorphology with nodular and plexiform patterns, may be multifocal, commonly metastasize to lymph nodes, often are resistant to imatinib, have unpredictable prognosis (indolent and protracted course) not related to size or mitotic rate, and may be syndromal associated with the Carney triad (GIST, extradrenal paraganglioma, and pulmonary chondroma) or Carney–Stratakis syndrome (GIST and familial paraganglioma); thus genetic testing for *SDH* mutations; particularly SDH-A should be done in these cases.

FNA Findings Smears show single or small clusters of plump or rounded epithelioid cells with a moderate amount of granular to clear cytoplasm, variable nuclear pleomorphism, bi- or multinucleation, and intranuclear inclusions (Fig. 5.9c–e). The nucleus is often pushed to an eccentric location. Large, bizarre cells may be found, but they carry no significance in the absence of high mitotic activity, large tumor size, and high nuclear grade. Of note, malignant epithelioid GISTs typically have small and more homogeneous cells.

The differential diagnosis includes mainly melanoma, endocrine neoplasm, extraadrenal paraganglioma, carcinoma, and lymphoma. For practical purposes, the diagnosis of GIST should be considered in aspirates of the GI tract, liver, mesentery, or abdominal-wall mass lesions when epithelioid cells are the predominant cell type. Large epithelioid malignant GISTs extending beyond the small-bowel wall must be differentiated by use of immunohistochemistry from large epithelioid sarcomas and sarcomatoid carcinomas arising in the kidney or retroperitoneum involving the intestinal wall (Fig. 5.10).

EUS Features The features are similar to those of spindle-cell GISTs.

Granular Cell Tumor

Granular cell tumors (GCTs) are reported to be the second most common esophageal mesenchymal tumors, after leiomyomas. These tumors, often benign, have a female predominance, are

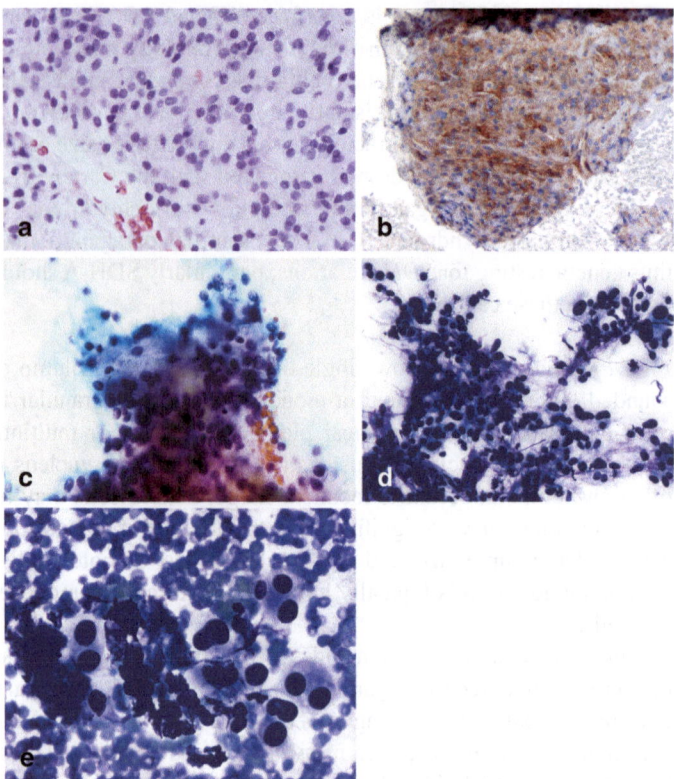

Fig. 5.9.   Gastrointestinal stromal tumor (*GIST*), epithelioid pattern. Histologic (**a**) and FNA (**c–e**) are similar to those of epithelial and nonepithelial neoplasms. Positive immunostain for CD117 (**b**) is helpful to make the
diagnosis. (**a**, H&E stain intermediate magnification; **b** Immunoperoxidase
stain for CD117; **c** Papanicolaou stain, high magnification; **d, e** DiffQuik
stain high magnification).

usually incidental findings, are particularly frequent in the distal
esophagus, and may be multicentric, both gastric and esophageal.
The tumor usually measures 1–2 cm and is submucosal and yellowish. Larger tumors may be circumferential and cause dysphagia.

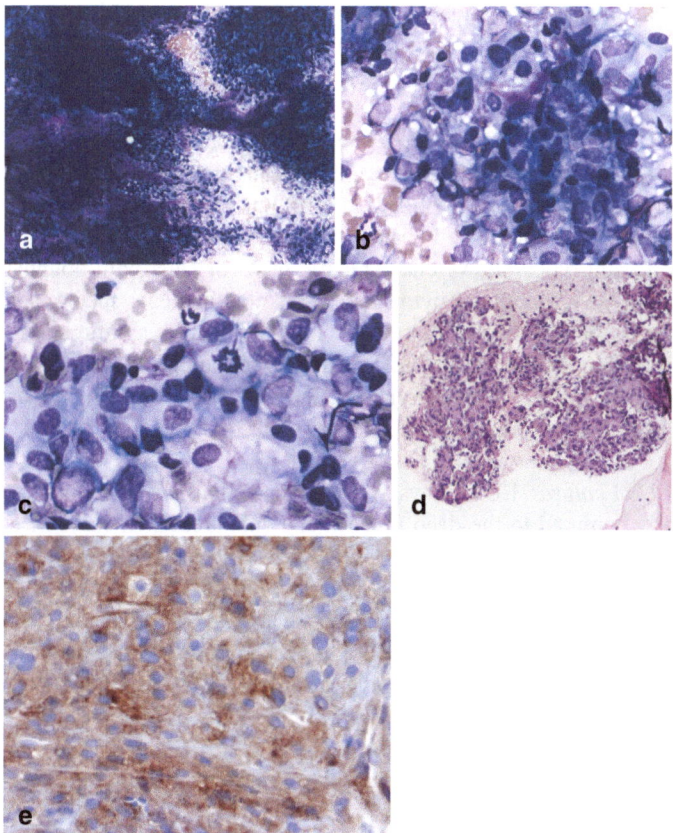

Fig. 5.10.   Malignant gastrointestinal stromal tumor (*GIST*). Epithelioid pattern-GIST with marked cellular pleomorphism and atypical mitotic figures resembling epithelioid sarcoma and poorly differentiated carcinoma (**a–d**). Immunostain for CD117 is positive (**e**). (**a–c** DiffQuik stain intermediate and high magnifications; **d**, H&E stain cell block; **e** Immunoperoxidase stain for CD117).

Histopathology Sections show nests of cells with granular and eosinophilic cytoplasm and round or elongated nuclei and occasional nucleoli (Fig. 5.11a). In the esophagus, the overlying epithelium may show pseudoepitheliomatous hyperplasia.

Immunoprofile Tumor is S-100 protein-, calretinin-, inhibin alpha-, nestin-, and CD68-positive. Tumor is also periodic acid-Schiff- (PAS) positive on diastase digestion (Fig. 5.11b).

FNA Findings Smears show sheets, clusters, and single cells with large round or spindle uniform, eccentrically placed nuclei. Purple granular cytoplasm is evident in DiffQuik-stained smears and can appear cyanophilic in Papanicolaou preparations (Figs. 5.11c, d). The cell block shows characteristic nests of cells with abundant granular eosinophilic cytoplasm and round nucleus; special stain for S-100 protein can be performed if necessary. Oxyntic cell hyperplasia may be mistaken for granular cell tumor; however, presence of chief cells in the vicinity and clinical correlation supports the non tumoral condition (Fig. 5.11e).

EUS Features EUS shows hypoechoic, smooth-edged lesions usually confined to the deep mucosa and submucosa. In cases of esophageal stricture, radial EUS may show a posterior heterogeneous submucosal esophageal mass invading the muscularis propria. By use of a high-frequency EUS probe, GCTs are found to be hyperechoic compared to the surrounding muscle layer in more than 50 % of cases. The GCTs have indistinct borders more frequently than do leiomyomas (Fig. 5.11f).

Heterotopic Pancreas

The prepyloric gastric antrum and duodenum around the common bile duct of adults and children are the most common sites for heterotopic pancreas, which may appear as an intramural nodule or a sessile polyp and be several centimeters in size. An esophageal location is exceedingly rare, although it may be more common in patients with trisomies 18 and 13. A characteristic endoscopic appearance, seen in 35 % of cases, demonstrates a raised subepithelial mound with central umbilication that represents the pancreatic duct (Fig. 5.12a). Conventional forceps biopsies may not be diagnostic.

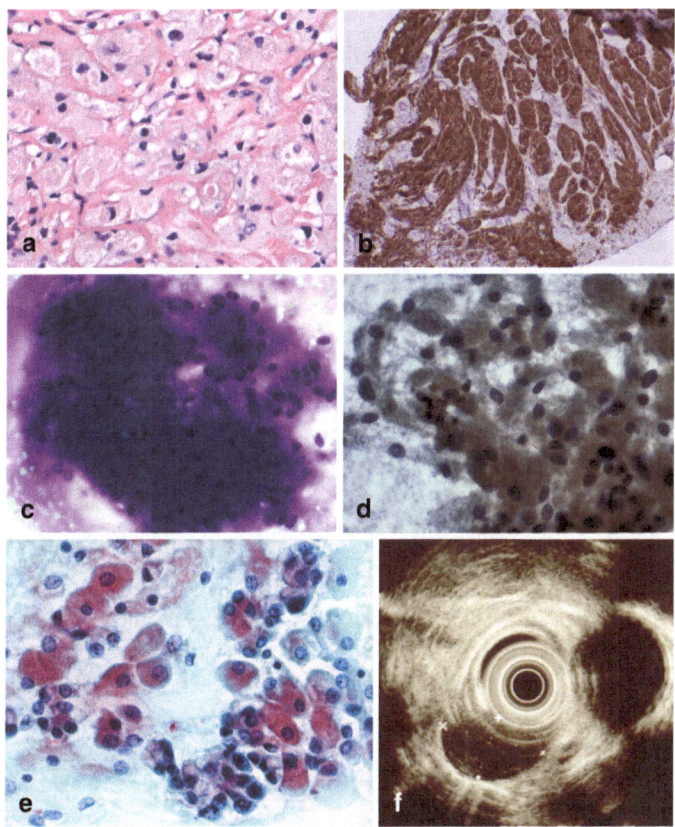

FIG. 5.11.   Granular cell tumor (*GCT*). A histologic section shows large cells with ample granular eosinophilic cytoplasm (**a**). Cells are S-100 protein positive (**b**). FNA smears show aggregates of cells with large and granular cytoplasm; the characteristic eosinophilic granules are best seen the Papanicolaou-stained smear (**c, d**). Oxyntic cells may be erroneously interpreted as granular cell tumor cells (**e**). Radial endoscopic ultrasound shows a hypoechoic well-circumscribed oval intramural mass (**f**). (**a**, H&E stain high magnification; **b** positive S-100 protein stain intermediate magnification; **c–e** DiffQuik and Papanicolaou stains high magnifications; **f** endoscopic ultrasound).

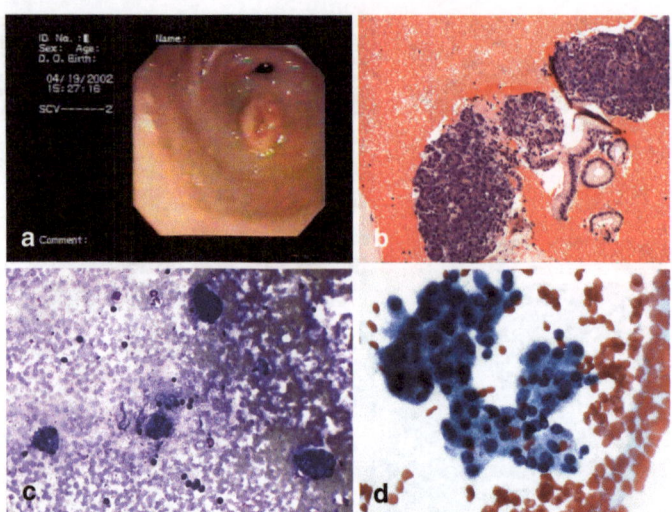

Fig. 5.12.   Heterotopic pancreas. Endoscopy shows a nodule with central umbilication in one-third of patients (**a**). Histologic and cytologic features of benign pancreatic acini are present in these mural nodules usually located in the gastric antrum. Sheets of pancreatic ductal epithelium may be seen. (**b**, H&E stain cell block intermediate magnification; **c** DiffQuik stain intermediate magnification; **d** Papanicolaou stain high magnification).

Histopathology The lesion is well demarcated and is located in the submucosa or muscularis propria. Pancreatic exocrine and endocrine elements in various proportions or ducts only, may be seen admixed with smooth-muscle bundles (Fig. 5.12b). Lesions and neoplasms arising in the various cellular elements have been described, i.e., pancreatitis, adenocarcinoma, cysts, and islet-cell tumors.

Immunoprofile Immunostain may not be necessary; however, endocrine markers such as chromogranin and synaptophysin, and exocrine markers such as trypsin, chymotrypsin, and alpha-amylase highlight the constituent cells.

FNA Findings EUS-FNA, when needed to exclude other diagnoses, shows a mixture of ductal and acinar elements (Figs. 5.12c, d).

However, some lesions may be largely cystic or composed of ducts only (adenomyoma), and a cytologic diagnosis may be difficult, if not impossible.

EUS Features On EUS, pancreatic rests are located predominantly in the submucosa, but may also involve the deep mucosa or muscularis propria. These lesions are predominantly hypoechoic (similar to normal pancreas tissue) and are typically heterogeneous. Anechoic duct-like structures may occasionally be seen in larger lesions. Characteristic EUS features of ectopic pancreas include indistinct borders, lobulated margins, the presence of anechoic duct-like structures, a mural growth pattern, and localization within two or more layers.

Brunner's Gland Lesions

Brunner's gland heterotopia is commonly small, rarely significant, and always located in the gastric antrum. Brunner's gland hyperplasia is commonly found incidentally in the duodenum, presents as multiple small nodules at endoscopy, and has no clinical significance.

Brunner's gland hamartoma, located in the submucosa and muscularis propria, can be hyperechoic, cystic, or solid and cystic on EUS and ulcerated on endoscopy, mimicking neoplasia. The hyperechoic appearance may mimic lipoma. It is often composed of multiple tissue types, including pancreatic tissue, and is surrounded by a fibrous capsule. Mucosal biopsies may be nondiagnostic, and EUS-FNA reveals glandular epithelium without atypia. If the lesion is located in the second portion of the duodenum, the differential diagnosis would include ampullary or periampullary well-differentiated adenocarcinoma.

GI Tract Lymphoma

Primary non-Hodgkin lymphomas (NHLs) of the GI tract are rare; however, the GI tract is the most common site of extranodal lymphoma. Esophageal lymphoma usually represents secondary extension of mediastinal Hodgkin or NHL or extension from a primary gastric NHL. Gastric NHL is the most common nonepithelial malignancy of the stomach and equally affects older individuals of both sexes. Diffuse large B-cell lymphoma (DLBCL) and extranodal marginal zone lymphoma (EMZL) are the most common subtypes found in the stomach.

Because these lesions are intramural, standard endoscopic biopsy may fail to obtain a diagnostic sample. In this instance, EUS-FNA with a 25-gauge needle is often sufficient for diagnosis and for triaging of specimens for flow cytometry, molecular diagnostics, immunohistochemistry, and cytogenetic studies. The definitive diagnosis of DLBCL can be made by these means; however, the diagnosis of EMZL may require the addition of an open biopsy for histomorphology. In addition to conventional diagnostic and staging procedures, EUS and EUS-FNA may allow preoperative determination of tumor and lymph-node classification. The cytomorphology and differential diagnosis are summarized in Tables 5.4 and 5.5.

Diffuse Large B-Cell Lymphoma (DLBCL)

This type of lymphoma occurs more frequently in the stomach than in other GI locations and may be primary or a transformation from EMZL; clear statistical data are not available. However, the clinical behavior of DLBCL and EMZL is similar. The lesion is unifocal, and most patients have a polypoid and ulcerative lesion. Regional lymph nodes are commonly involved at the time of diagnosis. *Helicobacter pylori* plays a role in DLBCL. The treatment of choice is chemotherapy followed by radiotherapy. DLBCL associated with EMZL may respond to antibiotic therapy; however, not as often as in pure EMZL. EUS is the most accurate method for local staging of gastric lymphoma, with 89% sensitivity, 97% specificity, and 95% overall accuracy for the evaluation of invasion depth.

Histopathology Similar to the finding in nodal DLBCL, there is diffuse infiltration of the GI wall by large lymphoid cells, i.e., sheets or aggregates of monomorphic immunoblasts or centroblasts with round or oval nuclei, scant cytoplasm, and variable nucleoli. Lymphoepithelial lesions may be seen particularly in cases associated with EMZL.

Immunoprofile DLBCL expresses a mature B-cell phenotype including CD19+ , CD20+ , CD22+ and CD79a+ cells with light chain restriction. CD5+ may suggest transformation from small lymphocytic lymphoma. BCL2, MUM-1, and BCL6+ are variably expressed.

Molecular Profile The most common abnormality involves the *BCL6* gene (*3q27*), followed by a *BCL2* translocation, t(14;18) (q32;q21). A few cases have *MYC* gene abnormalities, making the distinction from Burkitt lymphoma difficult.

FNA Findings Smears are cellular and show a predominant monotonous population of lymphoid cells of either large or intermediate size admixed with variable numbers of small lymphocytes and histiocytes and lymphoglandular bodies (Fig. 5.13a, b). Centroblasts are medium to large cells with scant cytoplasm, round or oval nuclei, often regular nuclear borders, and peripherally placed nucleoli. Immunoblasts are large cells with variable eosinophilic cytoplasm, round nuclei, and a prominent central nucleolus. Pleomorphic cells are seen in the anaplastic variant. The differential diagnosis is listed in Table 5.4.

EUS Features EUS shows significant hypoechoic thickening of the gastric wall, with a variable heterogeneous echotexture (Fig. 5.13c, d). The gastric layers are typically obliterated, and there may be extension of the lymphoma beyond the wall. Regional enlarged round deeply hypoechoic lymph nodes with well-defined margins are often present.

Perivascular Epithelioid Cell Tumor

Perivascular epithelioid cell tumor or PEComa is defined by coexpression of melanoma and muscle markers. PEComa is part of a group of tumors that include lymphangiomyolipoma,

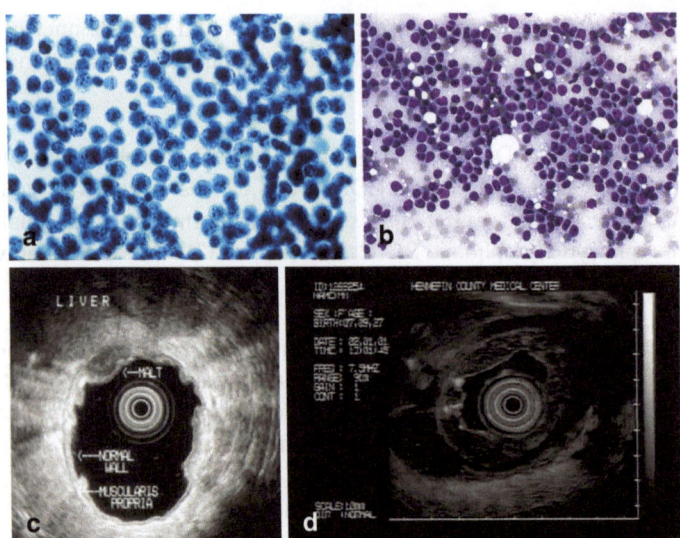

FIG. 5.13.   Non-Hodgkin lymphoma (*NHL*). Diffuse large B-cell lymphoma shows a monomorphic population of large cells with irregular nuclei and multiple nucleoli (**a**). Monomorphic intermediate size lymphoid cells with irregular nuclear contours are seen in this NHL (**b**). Endoscopic ultrasound shows focal (**c**) and diffuse (**d**) involvement of the gastric wall with obliteration of the layers. (**a, b** Papanicolaou and DiffQuik stains, high magnification).

angiomyolipoma, and clear-cell myomelanocytic "sugar" tumor. This tumor may arise in intraabdominal and somatic soft tissues and organs, including mainly the uterus and GI tract of adults, with female predominance. Most tumors follow a benign clinical course and rare ones recur or metastasize (Fig. 5.14a).

Histopathology Cells with epithelioid, spindle, or less commonly pleomorphic morphology are arranged in nests. Cells have clear or granular eosinophilic cytoplasm, vesicular nuclei, and prominent nucleoli and are surrounded by thin-walled vessels. Atypia, pleomorphism, mitosis, and necrosis may indicate an aggressive behavior with metastatic behavior (Fig. 5.14b–d).

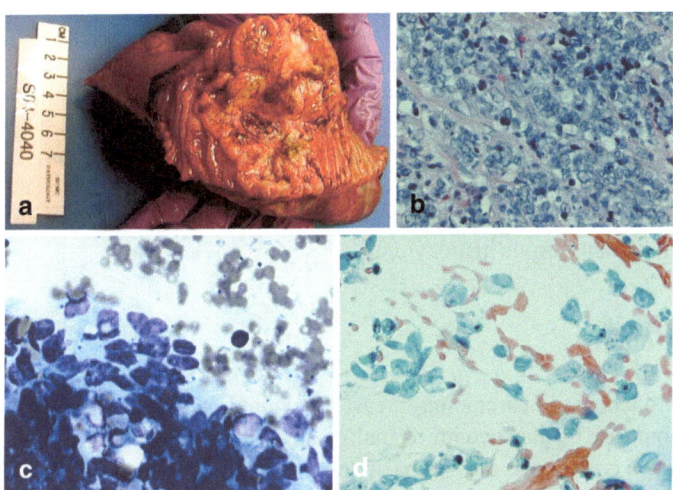

Fɪɢ. 5.14.   PEComa, malignant. This pleomorphic malignancy occurred in a 31-year-old woman who had a 12-cm jejunoileal tumor (**a**) with mesenteric lymph node metastasis. Tissue sections showed a pleomorphic malignancy (**b**). Smears showed large epithelioid pleomorphic cells (**c, d**) that stained positive for HMB45 and negative for S-100 protein, characteristic of this tumor. (**a** macroscopic feaures of the jejunal tumor; **b**, H&E stain high magnification; **c, d** DiffQuik and Papanicolaou stains high magnification).

Immunoprofile The pattern of SMA and HMB45 positivity is crucial for the diagnosis. More than 50 % are Melan-A-positive, and 25 % are desmin-positive. Cathepsin K may be a useful PEComa marker. Positivity with S-100 protein may be seen in rare instances.

Molecular Profile PEComas may show deletion or loss of chromosome 16p with inactivation or loss of *TSC2* gene (*TSC2* gene is located in chromosome 16p) that leads to inactivation of the mTOR pathway. Patients with metastatic PEComa may benefit from targeted therapy using rapamycin, also known as sirolimus against mTOR pathway.

Sarcomas with Epithelioid Characteristics

The involvement of the GI tract by these tumors can be primary or secondary by direct extension and must be in the differential diagnosis of epithelioid GIST. The list of potential sarcomas involving the GI tract includes (but is not restricted to) synovial sarcoma, epithelioid sarcoma, alveolar soft part sarcoma, angiosarcoma, and malignant fibrous histiocytoma.

Metastasis

Bronchogenic carcinoma, breast carcinoma, and malignant melanoma are the most common malignancies metastatic to the GI tract, most commonly the stomach. Ovarian cancer metastatic to the stomach and prostate cancer manifesting as metastatic perirectal mass have also been diagnosed by EUS-FNA.

The Epithelioid Small-Cell Pattern (Table 5.5)

Distinctions among these neoplasms are based principally on the characteristic immunoreactivity of these tumors. Endocrine marker positivity helps in the diagnosis of endocrine tumors. Usually more discohesive cells are seen in malignant lymphoma, and a B-cell phenotype identified by FCM will support the diagnosis. Epithelioid GIST may show small epithelioid cells and exhibits DOG-1, CD117, and CD34 positivity. Glomus tumor (actin +) and Hemangiopericytoma should also be considered in the differential diagnosis (vimentin +, keratin weak +). Some of these entities will be covered next.

Neuroendocrine Tumors (NETs)

The grastroenteropancreatic (GEP) tract is the most frequent site of NETs, followed by the bronchopulmonary system. Gastrointestinal (GI) NETs are divided by their embryonic origin into foregut (stom-

TABLE 5.5. The epithelioid small-cell pattern: cytology and immunohistochemistry.

Endocrine tumor	Epithelioid GIST	Glomus tumor	Lymphoma
Aggregates and single cells (usually small). Rosettes. Moderate cytoplasm. Salt-and-pepper chromatin	Aggregates and single cells (usually large). Granular chromatin. Abundant cytoplasm	Aggregates and single cells. Homogeneous and hyperchromatic nuclei	Single cells. Nuclei are monomorphic, round or irregular. Minimal cytoplasm. Variable nucleoli
Chromogranin (+) Synaptophysin (+) NSE (+). Keratin (+)	DOG-1 (+) CD117 (+) CD34 (+)	CD117(−). Actin (+), calponin (+), h-caldesmon (+), Vimentin (+)	B- and T-cell markers. Usually B-cell immunophenotype. Light chain restriction

GIST gastrointestinal stromal tumor

ach and duodenum), midgut (from duodenum beyond the Treitz ligament to the proximal transverse colon), and hindgut (distal colon and rectum). Ileal, appendiceal, cecal, and colorectal NETs are much more common than gastroduodenal ones. The main histologic categories of NETs of the GEP tract proposed by the WHO and the European Neuroendocrine Tumor Society (ENETS) are based on the degree of tumor differentiation and include low-grade (G1) and intermediate-grade (G2) grouped as well-differentiated NETs, and high-grade (G3) or poorly-differentiated neuroendocrine carcinomas (small cell or large cell). The classification is based on the mitotic count per ten HPF and Ki67 (proliferation marker) index (G1, <2 mitoses/ 10 hpf and Ki67 index <3%; G2, 2–10 mitoses/ 10 HPF or Ki67 index 3–20%; G3, >10 mitoses/ 10 HPF or Ki67 index >20%). It is advisable that, when this nomenclature is used in the cytology report, an explanatory note that includes other terminologies should be included e.g., "well-differentiated NET (carcinoid tumor)." According to American Joint Committee on Cancer (AJCC) guidelines, tumor staging for GI NETs depends on the location of the tumor, i.e., foregut, midgut, or hindgut. For

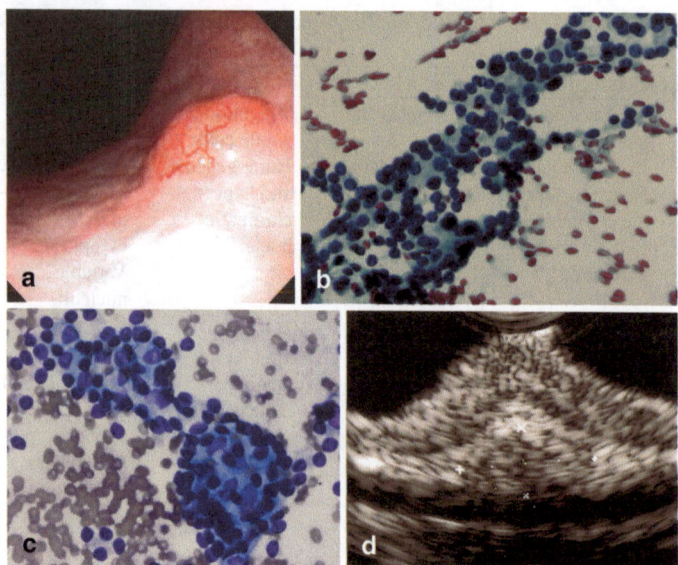

Fɪɢ. 5.15.   Gastric and duodenal neuroendocrine tumors. Macroscopic appearance of a gastric carcinoid (**a**) and FNA smear cytologic appearance of a duodenal gastrinoma (**b, c**). Endoscopic ultrasound appearance of the gastric carcinoid (**d**) with obliteration of layer 3 of the gastric wall. (**b, c** Papanicolaou and DiffQuik stains high magnification).

foregut and midgut NETs, T1 tumors measure ≤1 cm and invade lamina propria or submucosa; T2 tumors measure >1 cm or invade muscularis propria; T3 tumors penetrate subserosa (gastric, jejunal, and ileal NETs) or invade pancreas or retroperitoneum (ampullary or duodenal NETs); T4 tumors invade serosa and beyond. For hindgut NETs, T1 tumors measure ≤2 cm and invade lamina propria or submucosa; T2 tumors invade muscularis propria or measure >2 cm with invasion of lamina propria or submucosa; T3 tumors penetrate subserosa or into nonperitonealized perirectal or pericolic tissue; T4 tumors invade peritoneum and beyond.

Gastric NETs (gastric carcinoid tumors) are rare (Fig. 5.15a) and are classified into three types:

Type 1 is the most common (65 %) and arises in the setting of autoimmune chronic atrophic gastritis (pernicious anemia) with destruction of acid and intrinsic-factor-producing oxyntic cells, which results in hypergastrinemia and gastric carcinoid tumor 1–18 years after the initial diagnosis of gastritis. Tumors are usually < 1 cm, multifocal, and located in the gastric fundus and body.

Type 2 comprises 15 % of gastric carcinoid tumors (gastrinoma) and is associated with the Zollinger–Ellison syndrome and MEN-1 syndrome. The gastrinoma causes hypergastrinemia. These tumors are more aggressive than type 1 carcinoids. The tumors are usually < 1 cm, multifocal, and located in the gastric fundus and body.

Type 3 gastric carcinoid tumors are sporadic, with no predisposing factor. These tumors tend to be solitary, large (> 2 cm), to be located in the prepyloric region, and to be more prone to local invasion and metastasis (NE carcinoma). Carcinoid syndrome is rare in gastric carcinoid tumors, and usually associated with type 3 carcinoid.

Duodenal NETs, which may present in the context of an MEN-1 syndrome, are intramural nodules; endoscopically, they can be confused with Brunner's gland hamartomas or gastric heterotopia. Gastrinomas (G-cell tumors) are functioning in one-third of cases (Zollinger–Ellison syndrome), are often multiple, and occur as small submucosal nodules in the proximal duodenum. Somatostatinomas (D-cell tumors), usually nonfunctioning, are often solitary, occur almost exclusively at or around the ampulla of Vater, and may be associated with von Recklinghausen's disease. Carcinoid syndrome is exceedingly rare in duodenal NETs. Small-cell carcinomas are exceedingly rare and almost always occur in the periampullary region.

Functioning duodenal NETs are of either low or high grade. High-grade NE carcinomas are histologically poorly differentiated. Low-grade NETs are histologically well-differentiated; functioning ones are of any size or nonfunctioning ones > 2 cm. Duodenal NETs are usually benign when they are ≤ 1 cm and located within the mucosa–submucosa.

Ileal NETs are more common than *jejunal NETs*, the ileum being the most common site in the gastroenteric tract. The majority produce serotonin. Liver and lymph node metastases are not uncommon, and they may cause carcinoid syndrome; carcinoid syndrome is not always associated with liver metastasis. Jejunoileal NETs are often multicentric, large (> 2 cm), and locally invasive in the wall and mesentery. The clinical course is unpredictable and is only correlated with size and local invasion; cytomorphology, mitotic activity, and growth pattern do not predict metastatic disease. Metastasis is the only feature differentiating between a benign and malignant NET.

Colorectal NETs range from the most common well-differentiated NETs (carcinoid tumors) to the rare poorly differentiated NE carcinoma (small-cell carcinoma) and can occur in patients with MEN-1 syndrome. Rectal NETs are more common than cecal NETs. Cecal lesions can reach a large size. Carcinoid syndrome is uncommon.

Histopathology Gastroenteric NETs show small, round monomorphic cells that are arranged in various growth patterns, i.e., insular or nested, trabecular, and acinar. Cells have centrally located nuclei, finely granular ("salt and pepper") chromatin, and inconspicuous or absent nucleoli. Characteristically, an acinar pattern and luminal psammoma bodies are often seen in somatostatinomas. Gastrinomas and jejunoileal NETs do not have a particular growth pattern. Anaplasia, mitoses, and necrosis may indicate an aggressive behavior. The main differential diagnosis includes glomus tumor and lymphoma, as listed in Table 5.5. A spindle cell pattern may be seen occasionally (Fig. 5.6c).

Immunoprofile Synaptophysin, chromogranin, neuron-specific enolase (NSE), and keratin are positive. PDX1+, TTF1(−), and CDX2(−) support a gastric or duodenal origin.

Molecular Profile Gene expression profiling and supervised machine learning have been tested for classification of small intestine NETs and prediction of metastases with promising results. A panel of markers such as transcript levels of the genes melanoma antigen family D2 (*MAGE-D2*), metastasis-associated 1 (*MTA1*), nucleosome assembly protein 1-like (*NAP1L1*), Ki-67 (a marker of proliferation), survivin, frizzled homolog 7 (*FZD7*), Kiss1 metastasis suppressor (*Kiss1*), neuropilin 2 (*NRP2*), and chromogranin A (*CgA*), have been implicated in tumorigenicity, metastasis, and hormone production, and could be used for defining primary small-intestine NETs and for predicting the development of metastases.

FNA Findings Smears show high cellularity, with tumor cells in sheets, papillary fragments, loose groups, rosettes, and dispersed usually in a clean background (Fig. 5.15b, c). Cells are of moderate size and have a pale or finely granular, scant to moderate cytoplasm, round to oval uniform nuclei, smooth nuclear borders, and a finely granular chromatin with a "salt-and-pepper" appearance. A prominent spindle-cell cytomorphology may be seen, similar to tumors described in the spindle-cell pattern section (Fig. 5.5a, b). Tumor cells show cytoplasmic secretory granules on electron microscopy.

EUS Features Sonographically, these tumors are homogenous, well-demarcated, and hypoechoic (like GISTs), but more commonly they are localized to the submucosal layer without attachment to the muscularis propria. However, they may occasionally involve the superficial and deep mucosal layers (Fig. 5.15d).

Glomus Tumor

Glomus tumors are rare and usually are benign, solitary neoplasms that arise from modified smooth muscle cells of the glomus body, a type of neuromyoarterial receptor that plays a role in the regulation of arterial blood flow. Rare examples of metastatic glomus tumors have been described. They usually occur in the dermis or subcutis of the extremities and rarely in visceral locations, most often in the stomach of adults, with female predominance. Synchronous glomus tumor and GIST of the stomach can occur, and EUS-FNA may provide adequate sampling for an accurate diagnosis (Fig. 5.16a). Ultrastructural examination reveals prominent pinocytotic vesicles lining the plasmalemma.

Histopathology The tumors are circumscribed; with a median size is 2.5 cm. The pattern is multinodular with tumor nodules separated by smooth-muscle bundles. The nodules are composed of sheets of

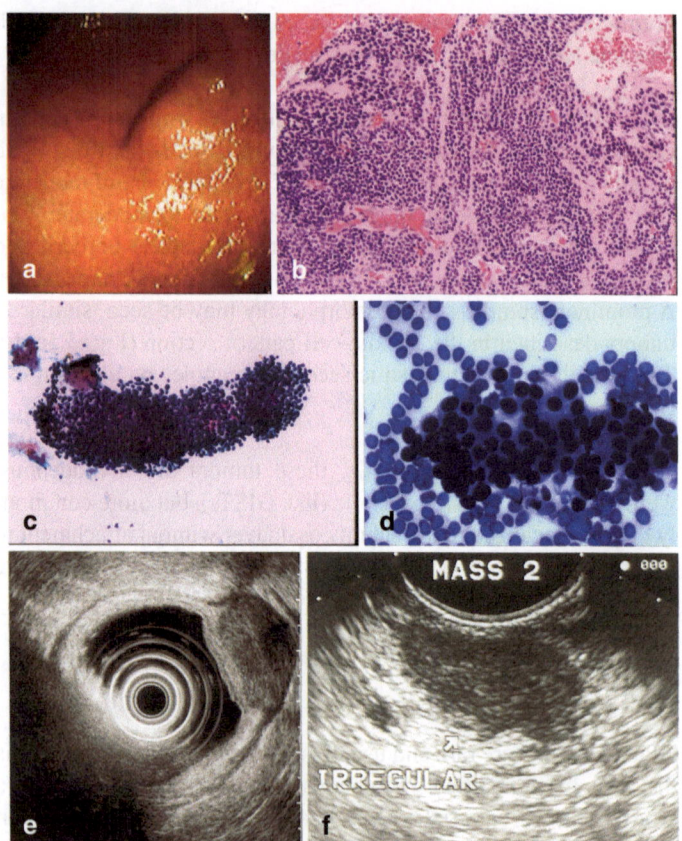

FIG. 5.16.   Glomus tumor. Endoscopic appearance of the intramural nodule in the stomach (**a**). Cell-block sections showing sheets of small uniform cells surrounding capillaries (**b**). Smears show fairly cohesive aggregates of small uniform cells with scant cytoplasm and round nuclei almost identical to those of neuroendocrine tumors (**c, d**). Endoscopic ultrasound appearance (**e** *radial*; **f** *linear*). (**b**, H&E stain intermediate magnification; **c, d** Papanicolaou and DiffQuik stains, high magnifications).

cells surrounded by capillaries (Fig. 5.16b). Cells are round with variably eosinophilic cytoplasm, well-defined cytoplasmic borders, and round, hyperchromatic, uniform nuclei.

Immunoprofile Immunohistochemical staining exhibits positivity for SMA, calponin, h-caldesmon, and vimentin, and negativity for desmin and CD117. Focal CD34 positivity may be seen in some cases. The differential diagnosis is listed in Table 5.5. Distinctions among these neoplasms are based principally on the characteristic immunoreactivity of these tumors. Hemangiopericytoma should also be considered in the differential diagnosis (vimentin+, keratin weak+).

Molecular Profile In addition to the protooncogene *RET* (associated with multiple endocrine neoplasia type 2, MEN-2) and the tumor-suppressor gene *VHL* (associated with von Hippel–Lindau disease), newly identified susceptibility genes for pheochromocytoma that include succinate dehydrogenase subunit D (*SDHD*) and succinate dehydrogenase subunit B (*SDHB*) are found. Their presence predisposes carriers to develop pheochromocytomas and glomus tumors.

FNA Findings Smears show groups of cohesive, uniform, and small, round to polygonal cells with scant cytoplasm, indistinct cell borders, and round, regular hyperchromatic nuclei with homogeneous chromatin (Fig. 5.16c, d).

EUS Features The EUS features of the lesion described include a sharply demarcated mass in the fourth layer of the gastric wall and a heterogeneous hypoechoic pattern with internal hyperechoic foci and a few tubular structures. We have previously encountered a case of synchronous glomus tumor and GIST. EUS showed two hypoechoic masses (Fig. 5.16e GIST and Fig. 5.16f glomus tumor), measuring 2.8 cm in greatest diameter each that appeared to arise from the muscularis propria. The glomus tumor had an irregular, slightly serrated extraluminal margin, possibly due to the increased vascular network (Figs 5.16f).

Extranodal Marginal Zone Lymphoma (EMZL)

The EMZL of mucosa-associated lymphoid tissue (MALT) is the most common type of lymphoma affecting the GI tract, particularly the stomach and small bowel. Gastric EMZL is usually multifocal, infiltrative, and larger than carcinoma, affects the antrum and body, and is associated with *H. pylori* infection. Treatment for *H. pylori* is effective in EMZL affecting the superficial mucosa (long-term remissions are seen in 70 % of low-grade EMZL). Tumors with *BCL-10* mutation and t(11;18) may not respond to this therapy. EUS is the most accurate method for local staging of gastric lymphoma, with 89% sensitivity, 97% specificity, and 95% overall accuracy for the evaluation of invasion depth.

Histopathology The lamina propria is expanded with a monotonous population of small- and medium-sized monocytoid cells admixed with immunoblasts and plasma cells. Lymphoepithelial lesions are seen as a result of the neoplastic invasion of gastric glands.

Immunoprofile Cells show a B-cell immunophenotype similar to that of marginal zone B-cells. CD20+ and CD43+ characterize the classic phenotype; however, CD43 is expressed in only 50% of cases. In these cases, IgH rearrangement by PCR supports the diagnosis. Flow cytometry or immunohistochemistry is useful for excluding follicular lymphoma (CD10+, BCL6+), small lymphocytic lymphoma (CD5+, and dim light-chain expression), and mantle cell lymphoma (CD5+, FMC7+).

Molecular Profile Chromosomal translocations found in EMZL and not in nodal marginal-zone lymphoma include: t(11;18) (q21;q21)/AP12-MALT1, t(1;14)(p22;q32)/IgH-BCL10, t(14;18) (q34;q21)/IgH-MALT1, and t(3;14)(p14.1;q32).

FNA Findings Monocytoid cells with gray cytoplasm, central nuclei, clumped chromatin, and small nucleoli are seen along with scattered larger transformed cells and plasma cells. The presence of numerous larger cells may indicate transformation to a large cell lymphoma.

EUS Features EUS show significant hypoechoic thickening of the gastric wall with a variable heterogeneous echotexture. The thickening may be limited to the mucosa, extend into the submucosa or, in more advanced cases the gastric layers are obliterated (Fig. 5.13c, d). There may be extension of the lymphoma beyond the wall. Regional enlarged, suspicious lymph nodes may be present. EUS demonstration of involvement of the submucosa or deeper layers predicts a low likelihood of regression following *H. pylori* eradication as a sole means of therapy.

Mantle Cell Lymphoma (MCL)

Thirty percent of nodal MCLs involve the GI tract, mainly the ileum of adults, with female predominance. Colonic and, less frequently, gastric and duodenal involvement is also seen. A single mass or multiple small nodules (lymphomatoid polyposis) may be seen in the GI tract, often associated with regional lymph-node involvement.

Histopathology There is a diffuse infiltrate of small lymphocytes with irregular nuclei and scant cytoplasm. A nodular pattern may also be seen. Mitoses are variable. Lymphoepithelial lesions are rare.

Immunoprofile The characteristic pattern is that of a mature B-cell phenotype with CD20+, CD5+, CD43+, BCL2+, CD10−, CD23−, and FMC7+. Nuclear cyclin D1 is almost always positive. Lambda light-chain restriction is commonly present. The differential diagnosis includes follicular lymphoma (CD10+, CD5−, cyclin D1−, BCL6+, BCL2+) and small lymphocytic lymphoma (CD10−, CD5+, CD23+, cyclin D1−, FMC7−), and EMZL (CD10−, cyclin D1−).

Molecular Profile The chromosomal translocation t(11;14) (q13;q32) between the *cyclin D1* gene and the *IGH* gene can be seen in almost all cases.

FNA Findings Smears show a monotonous population of small to intermediate-size lymphocytes similar to enterocytes with irregular nuclear contours, moderate amounts of slightly basophilic

cytoplasm, and inconspicuous nucleoli. Centroblasts, immunoblasts, or paraimmunoblasts are absent. Mitosis may be present.

Burkitt Lymphoma (BL)

This high-grade lymphoma in its three clinical forms (endemic,
sporadic, and immunodeficiency-associated) often occurs in extranodal sites including the GI tract. The Epstein–Barr virus (EBV)
genome is present in the neoplastic cells in all endemic cases and
is variably present in the other clinical forms. The endemic form
is a disease of childhood and usually involves the jaw and orbit;
the GI involvement is usually ileocecal. The sporadic form affects
children and young adults and involves the ileocecal area and rectum. The immunodeficiency associated with BL is often seen with
HIV infection.

Histopathology At low power, BL shows a characteristic "starry
sky" appearance with numerous medium-sized lymphocytes, a
round nucleus with several nucleoli, basophilic cytoplasm, and numerous small cytoplasmic vacuoles. Numerous mitoses and tingible body macrophages are present.

Immunoprofile Tumor cells express light-chain restriction and B-
cell-associated antigens. BCL2 is negative and BCL6 is positive.
The proliferation marker Ki-67 is positive in 100% of cells.

Molecular Profile MYC oncogene translocation at chromosome
segment 8q24 to the heavy chain gene at chromosome segment
14q32 t(8;14) without *BCL2* or *BCL6* translocation is almost always present.

FNA Findings Smears show a monotonous population of small to
intermediate-size lymphocytes with round nuclei, small nucleoli, and
a moderate amount of basophilic cytoplasm with lipid-containing
vacuoles 1–2 µm in size. Mitoses are numerous, and tingible body
macrophages are also present. Plasmacytoid or pleomorphic cells
may be present, particularly in immunodeficiency-associated cases.

Enteropathy-Associated T-cell Lymphoma

This rare type of lymphoma is seen in association with gluten enteropathy and affects adults, with no gender predilection. Most patients have localized intestinal disease and rarely have multiorgan involvement. Tissue sections show a monotonous population of small to medium-sized lymphocytes with irregular nuclear contours and conspicuous nucleoli. Eosinophils and histiocytes are also present. Medium-size, pleomorphic, and anaplastic (CD30+, ALK1 −) forms have been described. Most cases are CD3+, CD4−, CD8−, CD7+, CD103+, CD5− and express cytotoxic granule-associated protein TIA-1.

The Cystic Pattern

Embryologic ectopia of the foregut or hindgut, consisting of any or all layers of the gut wall, may give rise to gut congenital cysts/duplications. In the esophagus, cysts may present in childhood and cause dysphagia, but many are asymptomatic and are detected incidentally in adulthood. Most are located in the lower third of the esophagus, and some are intramural, whereas others are extrinsic.

Duplication cysts (most commonly found to be associated with the esophagus) characteristically have a duplicated muscularis propria and are lined by columnar ciliated, squamous, gastric, or enteric epithelium. Gastric duplication cysts are rare (2–4 %), mostly located in the greater curvature and pylorus, discovered incidentally at upper GI endoscopy, and are round or ovoid (Fig. 5.17a).

EUS and EUS-FNA can be used for diagnosing these cysts, avoiding surgery with its associated morbidity. On EUS, they form a compressible structure in the submucosa and are generally anechoic with posterior acoustic enhancement (Fig. 5.17b, c). Cysts may contain thick, viscous mucus with suspended debris, in which case they are hypoechoic, rather than anechoic. In this scenario, the sonographic appearance may be confused with GIST or other mesenchymal tumors; however needle aspiration will readily

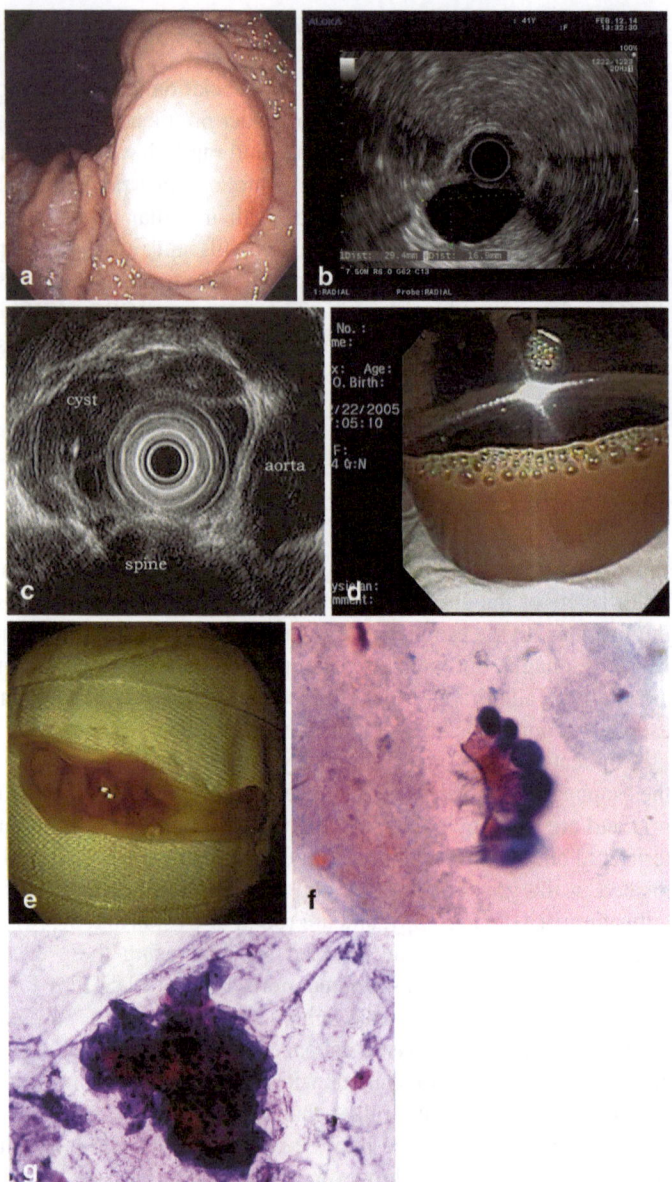

FIG. 5.17.   Endoscopic (**a**) and EUS view (**b**) of a trilobed gastric body cyst showing posterior acoustic enhancement. Endoscopic ultrasound im-

demonstrate the liquid nature of the contents (Fig. 5.17d, e). Duplication cysts may have sonographically-identifiable wall layers resembling normal mucosa, submucosa and muscularis propria. The identification of distinct wall layers is characteristic and diagnostic.

Because gastric cysts are commonly lined by gastric epithelium, the cytologic evaluation of may be equivocal; likewise, esophageal cysts lined by squamous cells may be difficult to be diagnosed cytologically without EUS needle placement correlation. On the contrary, cysts with respiratory-type epithelium, most likely of a developmental type, can be diagnosed unequivocally by EUS-FNA (Figs. 5.17f, g). The demonstration of detached ciliary tufts in the cyst fluid is helpful for the diagnosis. Foregut cysts have also been described in the mediastinal cysts section of this book.

On EUS, bronchogenic cysts are anechoic and are found in the submucosa. They are rarely found in the stomach. Bronchogenic cysts do not have sonographically identifiable wall layers within the cyst wall.

Thick Gastric Folds

Hypertrophic gastric folds, endoscopically defined as prominent rugal folds that fail to be obliterated with insufflation, are seen in various benign and malignant conditions (Fig. 5.18a). The differential diagnosis for this endoscopic finding includes a variety of malignant conditions such as lymphoma and diffusely infiltrative signet ring carcinoma, granulomatous processes (Crohn's disease, sarcoidosis, syphilis, anisakiasis), mucosal hyperplasia (Menetrier's disease, Zollinger–Ellison syndrome), acute gastric mucosal lesion, acute or severe gastritis (*H. pylori* lymphocytic

---

age of an esophageal cyst showing reduplicated wall (**c**) and an anechoic intramural mass. A thin brown chocolate color fluid (**d**) and thick mucus (**e**) are the gross appearances of a gastric and esophageal cyst respectively. Presence of ciliated epithelial cells is diagnostic (**f**); however the presence of squamous cells (**g**) in esophageal cysts or glandular cells in gastric cysts needs clinical end EUS correlation. (**f, g** Papanicolaou stain high magnifications).

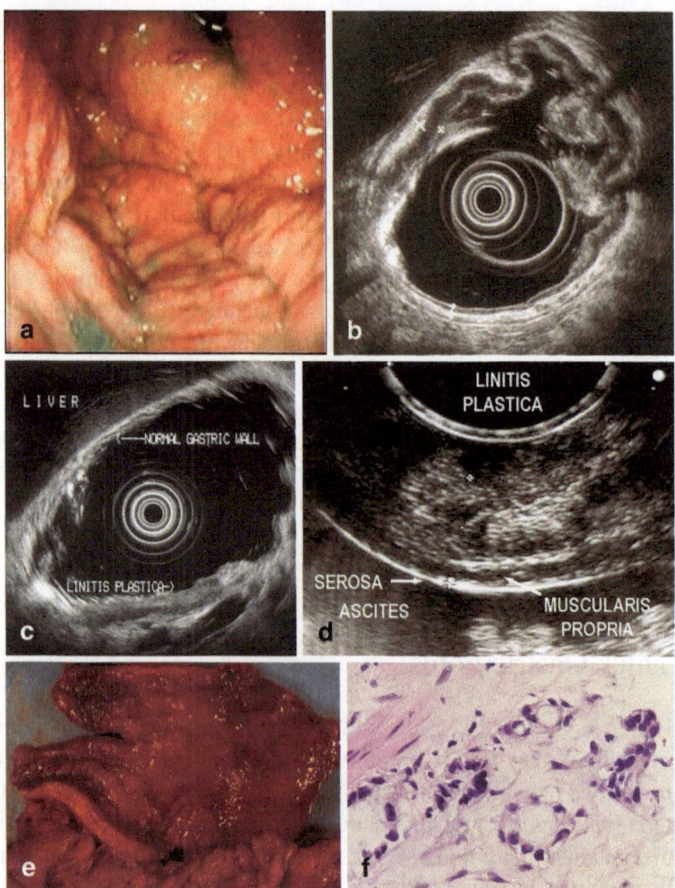

Fig. 5.18.   Thick gastric folds as seen endoscopically (**a**). Endoscopic ultrasound radial view of a case of Menetrier's disease (**b**). There is marked
thickening of layer 2 (deep mucosa) but preservation of the normal five-
layered echostructure. In contrast, the sonographic appearance of linitis
plastica (**c**—radial, **d**—linear) shows hypoechoic tissue which infiltrates
layers 2, 3, and 4 with a loss of distinct tissue planes. Gross, histologic and
cytologic features seen in smears from gastric adenocarcinoma, signet ring
cell type (**e–g**). A small pocket of malignant ascites (**h**) was sampled with
cytology positive for adenocarcinoma (**i**). (**f**, H&E stain high magnification; **g** and **i** DiffQuik stain high magnifications).

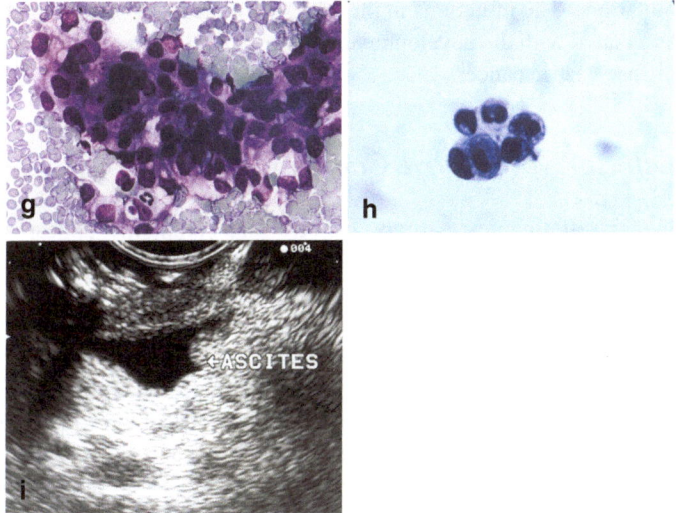

F<small>IG</small>. 5.18.   (continued)

or cytomegaloviral (CMV)), and eosinophilic gastroenteritis. Although the EUS appearance may often suggest a specific diagnosis, malignant conditions such as lymphoma (Fig. 5.13d) and carcinoma, either primary or metastatic, causing linitis plastica require pathologic correlation (Figs. 5.18b–d).

Gastric adenocarcinoma is the second most common cause of cancer in the world, the most common gastric epithelial neoplasia, and can be divided in intestinal and diffuse types (Lauren classification). Cancer arising in the gastroesophageal junction (GEJ) and gastric cardia within 5 cm from the GEJ is now classified as esophageal. The risk factors associated with the development of gastric cancer include environmental (diet, smoking), chronic gastritis-related intestinal metaplasia (for the intestinal-type more than for the diffuse-type of gastric cancer), and *H. pylori* infection (for both cancer types), particularly if present for more than 10 years prior to diagnosis of cancer. Most gastric cancers occur sporadically; however, some genetic alterations have been linked to the development of gastric cancer, i.e., Li-Fraumeni syndrome, familial adenomatous polyposis, hereditary nonpolyposis colon cancer, and *BRCA2* mutations. The mutations in the adhesion molecule E-cadherin are associated with the development of autosomal dominant hereditary diffuse gastric cancer.

Diffuse-Type Gastric Carcinoma

In contrast to intestinal-type cancers that commonly appear as polypoid, fungating, and ulcerated masses, the diffuse-type cancer may appear infiltrating or depressed with no obvious mucosal mass or lesion. As such, these tumors often appear endoscopically as thickened gastric folds. Linitis plastic is rare, and describes the thick-, firm-, leathery-appearing gastric wall infiltrated by diffuse-type carcinoma (Fig. 5.18e). Whereas carcinomas of intestinal type are usually readily visualized endoscopically and diagnosed by standard forceps biopsies, standard biopsy results are often inconclusive in diffuse-type carcinomas. EUS is unique in its ability to image tumor extension in the gastric wall very precisely and aids in obtaining a definitive pathologic diagnosis via EUS-FNA or EUS-guided core biopsy.

Histopathology Diffuse-type adenocarcinomas of the distal esophagus, rectum, and more commonly of the stomach have predominantly an intramural infiltrative pattern and they elicit a desmoplastic stromal reaction that results in wall rigidity, thickening, and lack of elasticity. Cells often have a signet ring cell appearance with variable intracytoplasmic mucin, which is less evident in poorly differentiated tumors (Fig. 5.18f). Linitis plastica may also be secondary to breast, prostate, and urothelial carcinomas that are metastatic to the stomach.

Immunoprofile Gastric adenocarcinoma is keratin, EMA-, CEA-, and mucin-positive. CK7 and CD20 are variable; however, CK7+ and CK20− are frequent.

Molecular Profile Diffuse-type gastric adenocarcinoma may be hereditary, and patients may have a germline *E-cadherin* mutation. Family members must be tested, and, if positive, a prophylactic gastrectomy is indicated because gastric adenocarcinoma may occur during the teenage years.

FNA Findings EUS-FNA cytology of adenocarcinoma exhibits scant cellularity, with singly dispersed and small groups of malignant cells that have prominent cytoplasmic mucinous vacuolization, eccentrically placed nuclei, coarse chromatin, and conspicuous nucleoli (Fig. 5.18g). Metastases to regional lymph nodes often occur and are amenable to EUS-FNA sampling and diagnosis. In the presence of malignant ascites, and in contrast to more revealing molecular tests performed on peritoneal fluid, the diagnosis of peritoneal carcinomatosis may not always be evident by cytology (Fig. 5.18h, i). Rarely, nonneoplastic conditions resulting in thickening of the gut wall can be diagnosed by EUS-FNA. Eosinophilic gastroenteritis is characterized by thickening of the stomach and small bowel because of infiltration by eosinophils.

EUS Features Characteristic sonographic findings of linitis include gastric-wall rigidity and a gastric wall thickness of >6 mm (double the normal gastric wall thickness of <3 mm). The mean thickness is 13 mm. There may be diffuse hypoechogenicity of the wall with loss of architecture or alternatively there may be focal prominence of the existing wall layers which become distended with swirls of hypoechoic material (Fig. 5.18d, i).

Sonographic Features of Thick Gastric Folds

The following sonographic features are useful in the differential diagnosis of thick gastric folds:

1. Gastric wall compressibility is preserved in benign conditions, is absent in gastric carcinoma, and may be preserved or absent in gastric lymphoma.
2. Echogenicity is variable. Gastric lymphoma shows the lowest echogenicity.

3. EUS identification of the thickened or affected gut layer(s) is a diagnostic clue. In acute gastric mucosal lesion (AGML) and anisakiasis, wall stratification is preserved, and the main thickened layer is the third layer (submucosa). In Menetrier's disease, the main thickened layer is the second layer (deep mucosa, muscularis mucosa), and wall stratification is preserved.
4. The wall thickness is similar in all disorders except AGML, in which it may be significantly less than that of anisakiasis, gastric lymphoma, and carcinoma.

Further Reading

Agaimy A, Wunsch PH. Gastrointestinal stromal tumours: a regular origin in the muscularis propria, but an extremely diverse gross presentation. A review of 200 cases to critically re-evaluate the concept of so-called extra-gastrointestinal stromal tumours. Langenbecks Arch Surg. 2006;391(4):322–9.

Agaimy A, Gaumann A, et al. Primary and metastatic high-grade pleomorphic sarcoma/malignant fibrous histiocytoma of the gastrointestinal tract: an approach to the differential diagnosis in a series of five cases with emphasis on myofibroblastic differentiation. Virchows Arch. 2007;451(5):949–57.

Agaimy A, Bihl MP, et al. Calcifying fibrous tumor of the stomach: clinicopathologic and molecular study of seven cases with literature review and reappraisal of histogenesis. Am J Surg Pathol. 2010;34(2):271–8.

Bardales RH, Stelow EB, et al. Review of endoscopic ultrasound-guided fine-needle aspiration cytology. Diagn Cytopathol. 2006;34(2):140–75.

Corless CL. Gastrointestinal stromal tumors: what do we know now? Mod Pathol. 2014;27(Suppl 1):1–16.

Debol SM, Stanley MW, et al. Glomus tumor of the stomach: cytologic diagnosis by endoscopic ultrasound-guided fine-needle aspiration. Diagn Cytopathol. 2003;28(6):316–21.

Dwight T, Benn DE, et al. Loss of SDHA expression identifies SDHA mutations in succinate dehydrogenase-deficient gastrointestinal stromal tumors. Am J Surg Pathol. 2013;37(2):226–33.

Edge SB. American Joint Committee on Cancer. AJCC Cancer Staging Manual. 7th ed. New York: Springer; 2010.

Fletcher CD, Berman JJ, et al. Diagnosis of gastrointestinal stromal tumors: a consensus approach. Hum Pathol. 2002;33(5):459–65.

Gomes AL, Bardales RH, et al. Molecular analysis of c-Kit and PDGFRA in GISTs diagnosed by EUS. Am J Clin Pathol. 2007;127(1):89–96.

Hawes RH. The evolution of endoscopic ultrasound: improved imaging, higher accuracy for fine needle aspiration and the reality of endoscopic ultrasound-guided interventions. Curr Opin Gastroenterol. 2010;26(5):436–44.

Huss S, Kunstlinger H, et al. A subset of gastrointestinal stromal tumors previously regarded as wild-type tumors carries somatic activating mutations in KIT exon 8 (p.D419del). Mod Pathol. 2013;26(7):1004–12.

Kirsch R, Gao ZH, et al. Gastrointestinal stromal tumors: diagnostic challenges and practical approach to differential diagnosis. Adv Anat Pathol. 2007;14(4):261–85.

Klimstra DS, Modlin IR, et al. Pathology reporting of neuroendocrine tumors: application of the Delphic consensus process to the development of a minimum pathology data set. Am J Surg Pathol. 2010;34(3):300–13.

Kodera Y, Nakanishi H, et al. Detection of disseminated cancer cells in linitis plastica-type gastric carcinoma. Jpn J Clin Oncol. 2004;34(9):525–31.

Liu TC, Lin MT, et al. Inflammatory fibroid polyps of the gastrointestinal tract: spectrum of clinical, morphologic, and immunohistochemistry features. Am J Surg Pathol. 2013;37(4):586–92.

Makhlouf HR, Ahrens W, et al. Synovial sarcoma of the stomach: a clinicopathologic, immunohistochemical, and molecular genetic study of 10 cases. Am J Surg Pathol. 2008;32(2):275–81.

Miettinen M. Smooth muscle tumors of soft tissue and non-uterine viscera: biology and prognosis. Mod Pathol. 2014;27(Suppl 1):17–29.

Miettinen M, Sarlomo-Rikala M, et al. Gastrointestinal stromal tumors and leiomyosarcomas in the colon: a clinicopathologic, immunohistochemical, and molecular genetic study of 44 cases. Am J Surg Pathol. 2000;24(10):1339–52.

Miettinen M, Makhlouf HR, et al. Plexiform fibromyxoma: a distinctive benign gastric antral neoplasm not to be confused with a myxoid GIST. Am J Surg Pathol. 2009;33(11):1624–32.

Mitteldorf CA, Birolini D, et al. A perivascular epithelioid cell tumor of the stomach: an unsuspected diagnosis. World J Gastroenterol. 2010;16(4):522–5.

Montgomery E. Tumors of the Esophagus. In: Iacobuzio-Donahue CA, Montgomery E, editors. Gastrointestinal and liver pathology. Philadelphia: Elsevier Saunders; 2012. pp. 35–64.

Nguyen T, Fisher C, et al. Gastrointestinal mesenchymal tumors. In: Iacobuzio-Donahue CA, Montgomery E, editors. Gastrointestinal and liver pathology. Philadelphia: Elsevier Saunders; 2012. pp. 208–56.

Okanobu H, Hata J, et al. Giant gastric folds: differential diagnosis at US. Radiology. 2003;226(3):686–90.

Park JY, Fenton HH, et al. Epithelial neoplasms of the stomach. In: Iacobuzio-Donahue CA, Montgomery E, editors. Gastrointestinal and liver pathology. Philadelphia: Elsevier Saunders; 2012. pp. 142–60.

Stelow EB, Stanley MW, et al. Endoscopic ultrasound-guided fine-needle aspi-
    ration findings of gastrointestinal leiomyomas and gastrointestinal stromal
    tumors. Am J Clin Pathol. 2003;119(5):703–8.
Stelow EB, Lai R, et al. Endoscopic ultrasound-guided fine-needle aspi-
    ration cytology of peripheral nerve-sheath tumors. Diagn Cytopathol.
    2004;30(3):172–7.
Stelow EB, Murad FM, et al. A limited immunocytochemical panel for the dis-
    tinction of subepithelial gastrointestinal mesenchymal neoplasms sampled
    by endoscopic ultrasound-guided fine-needle aspiration. Am J Clin Pathol.
    2008;129(2):219–25.

Chapter 6
ERUS and ERUS-FNA of Intramural and Extramural Masses of the Colorectum

Zahra Maleki

General Considerations

Introduction

Endoscopic ultrasonography (EUS), first introduced into clinical practice in 1980, is a combination of endoscopy and intraluminal sonography. With use of high-frequency transducers, endorectal endoscopic ultrasound (ERUS) allows highly detailed assessment of the rectal-wall layers as well as visualization of the extraluminal structures (Fig. 6.1). ERUS is used routinely in clinical practice for diagnosis and staging of malignancies of the colorectum, prostate, bladder, and female genital tract. ERUS is highly accurate for distinguishing between benign tumors and invasive carcinomas, and between tumors localized to the rectal wall and those with transmural invasion. New techniques that have contributed significantly to the evolution of ERUS include three-dimensional ERUS, use of high-frequency miniprobes, transrectal ultrasound-guided biopsy techniques, and hydrogen peroxide-enhanced endosonography. Curved-linear-array echoendoscopes use an electronic transducer

Z. Maleki (✉)
Department of Pathology, Division of Cytopathology, The Johns Hopkins Hospital, 600 N. Wolfe Street, PATH 406, Baltimore, MD 21287-6940, USA
e-mail: zmaleki1@jhmi.edu

R. H. Bardales (ed.), *Cytology of the Mediastinum and Gut Via Endoscopic Ultrasound-Guided Aspiration,* Essentials in Cytopathology 25,
DOI 10.1007/978-3-319-12796-5_6,
© Springer International Publishing Switzerland 2015

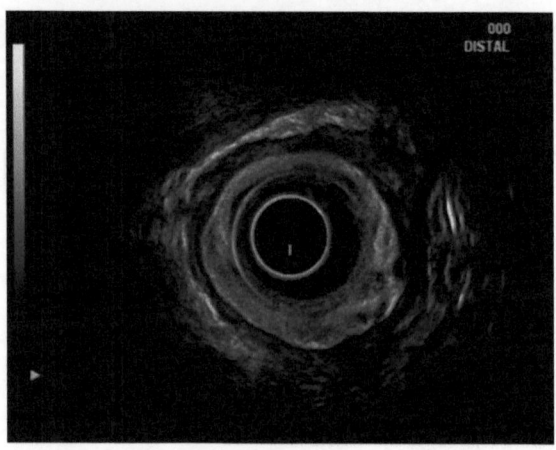

FIG. 6.1. Radial EUS showing the five circumferential layers of the normal rectal wall. (Courtesy of Drs. Vikesh K. Singh and Vivek Kumbhari, The Johns Hopkins Hospital, Maryland, USA).

and offer the ability to perform interventional procedures such as fine-needle aspiration (FNA).

ERUS-FNA, developed in the early 1990s, enhances the diagnostic yield of ERUS by providing material for microscopic evaluation. The diagnostic yield of ERUS-FNA has been reported to be 89–96%, whereas, the success rate for imaging investigation alone without histologic findings was 81.8%. The overall sensitivity, specificity, and positive and negative predictive values of ERUS-FNA are reported to be 89% (74–100%), 79% (50–100%), 89% (74–100%), and 79% (51–100%), respectively. FNA especially improves the accuracy of ERUS in the diagnosis of recurrent rectal cancer.

Rapid on-site evaluation of the aspirated material by a cytopathologist or cytotechnologist for specimen adequacy increases the diagnostic yield. Specimens obtained by ERUS-FNA can easily be processed for cytologic diagnosis and for ancillary tests including, but not limited to, immunostains, cultures, flow cytometry, or molecular studies.

ERUS-FNA Procedure

ERUS- FNA is usually well tolerated, with conscious sedation providing increased comfort. The procedure can be performed by a gastroenterologist or radiologist in either the endoscopy or the ultrasound unit on an outpatient basis. ERUS is preferably performed on a clean, empty rectum. Laxative enemas are usually sufficient; however standard colonoscopy preparation optimizes imaging. A rigid probe or a flexible echoendoscope with a radial transducer is used for ultrasound examination of intraluminal rectal lesions. A linear transducer is routinely used when FNA sampling is needed. The bowel wall is seen under ERUS as five alternating hyper- and hypoechoic layers. Informed consent is obtained after the risks and benefits of the procedure are explained to the patient.

The patient is placed in the left lateral decubitus position. Administered medications, oxygenation, and vital signs are monitored constantly during the procedure. A colonoscopy is performed for the direct visualization of the mucosa. Subsequently, ERUS with the use of a high-frequency radial-imaging echoendoscope is done. Water is used as necessary to provide an adequate acoustic interface. After the lesion is detected, measurements are documented and ERUS-FNA is performed as described for EUS-FNA of the upper digestive tract in Chap. 2. Color Doppler ultrasound is used for identifying and avoiding any vessels.

The Role of the Cytopathologist or Cytotechnologist

A cytopathologist or cytotechnologist evaluates the aspirated material on-site. The number of passes and specimen triage are determined by cytology findings on-site. In most cases of solid masses, three or more passes are performed. Needle rinses and clotted blood are transferred to the transport medium or formalin as needed for making cell blocks and possible further ancillary tests. Flow-cytometry studies are done on aspirated material when the cytology findings are suspicious for lymphoma on immediate interpretation. Material is sent to the microbiology laboratory for cultures when the cytology findings indicate an infectious process. In the case of benign cystic lesions or abscess, on- site evaluation allows the endoscopist to aspirate the fluid and drain the cyst or abscess.

Indications

ERUS-FNA is a safe and efficient method used in clinical practice for evaluation of any suspicious intramural, extramural, and or perirectal mass lesions by providing cytology material for microscopic examination. ERUS-FNA is used for evaluation of (1) the depth of transmural invasion in colorectal cancer; (2) tumor staging of colorectal, anal, and other locoregional cancers; (3) tumor invasion of perirectal fat; (4) nodal status and nodal metastasis; (5) suspected recurrent cancers in and adjacent to surgical anastomoses; (6) tumor recurrence or metastasis; (7) the presence of malignancy before chemotherapy, radiation therapy, and/or aggressive surgery; (8) pelvic masses; (9) intramural and submucosal masses; and (10) perirectal cystic masses.

Contraindications

Contraindications include the inability to clearly visualize a lesion or a tumor mass, or presence of a vessel interposed in the path between the needle and the target.

Complications

The complication rate is 1–2%, which is similar to that of computed tomography (CT) or percutaneous ultrasound-guided FNA. The major reported complications are infections in cystic lesions, and bleeding. Most reported complications are from EUS-FNA of upper gastrointestinal tract or pancreas. Bacteremia occurs after ERUS-FNA at a rate similar to that of colonoscopy, but it does not warrant the prophylactic administration of antibiotics. Occasionally, prophylactic antibiotics are prescribed, depending upon the patient's general condition. The risk of tumor seeding along the biopsy tract is very small, with only rare anecdotal cases reported.

The Role of ERUS-FNA in Colorectal Cancer Staging

The prognosis of rectal cancer correlates with pathologic staging at the time of diagnosis. ERUS has become the method of choice for locoregional colorectal cancer staging.

ERUS is the most accurate modality for assessing the local depth of invasion into the rectal-wall layers (T staging in the TNM classification); the prefix "u" is suggested in T staging by use of an ultrasound. ERUS can detect early cancers, residual carcinoma in the rectal wall, and local recurrence at an anastomosis site.

For nodal (N) staging, involvement is usually suspected if a lymph node is round, hypoechoic, and >5 mm in diameter, features which may differentiate it from a non-neoplastic node. ERUS alone is not as accurate for predicting nodal metastasis as it is for tumor depth. Preoperative ERUS-FNA may enhance the identification of extra-mesenteric lymph node metastasis outside a standard radiation field or mesorectal resection margin, and it may affect the choice of surgical or chemoradiation treatment strategy.

Accurate preoperative staging determines both the type of surgery performed and the decision to use neoadjuvant therapy. Inaccurate staging tends to result from over-staging because of associated (1) peri-tumoral inflammation; (2) difficulty distinguishing malignant from reactive lymphadenopathy; (3) chemoradiation effects such as inflammation, edema, necrosis, or fibrosis; and (4) postradiation changes such as fibrosis that is difficult to distinguish from residual tumor. Preservation of the anal sphincter is the goal in treatment of patients who have low-lying, locally advanced rectal cancer, because it decreases morbidity and improves the quality of life. Preoperative chemoradiation in these patients improves local control and is associated with an increased rate of sphincter preservation. Complete tumor staging is compromised in approximately 14% of patients because of luminal tumor stenosis.

Comparative studies have demonstrated that the accuracy of ERUS T and N colorectal cancer staging is superior to that of CT and equivalent to that of MRI. Overall, ERUS accuracy in numerous studies ranges from 80 to 95 % for T-staging and from 70 to 75 % for N-staging. These levels are slightly higher than the 75–85 % for T staging and 60–70 % for N-staging for MRI and 65–75 % and 55–65 %, respectively, for helical CT.

A succinct description of the most common intra- and extramural masses of the colorectum evaluated and diagnosed by ERUS and ERUS-FNA are covered in the next sections.

ERUS-FNA of Benign Intramural Colorectal Masses

Leiomyoma

Leiomyoma of the colorectum is a rare benign tumor arising from the muscularis layer of the colorectal wall of adults, predominantly males with a median age of 60 years. It presents as a well-delineated, white, and firm polypoid nodule. A conservative excision is therapeutic.

Histopathology The tumor is a well-circumscribed submucosal mass consisting of benign appearing smooth-muscle cells. Necrosis and atypical mitoses are not features of leiomyoma, whereas nuclear pleomorphism can be seen.

Immuno-Profile The tumor cells are immunoreactive for smooth muscle actin and desmin and non-reactive for CD117, S-100 protein, and CD34.

FNA Findings Aspirated material of ERUS-FNA is usually scant. It consists of benign-appearing, spindled smooth-muscle cells arranged mainly in tissue fragments (Fig. 6.2). Necrosis, atypical mitoses, or nuclear pleomorphism is not seen. Diagnostic immuno-histochemistry can be done on the cell blocks.

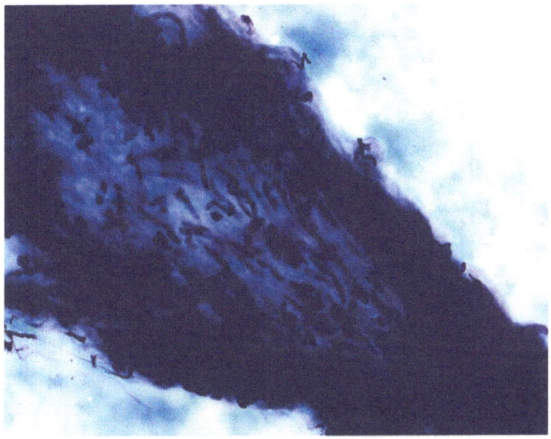

Fig. 6.2. Leiomyoma. Tissue fragment showing cohesive spindle cells with ill-defined cytoplasmic borders, elongated nuclei with blunt ends, and a dense, glassy stroma (DiffQuik stain, X400).

ERUS Features A well-defined, homogeneous hypoechoic intramural mass, often originating from the muscularis propria, is identified.

Lipoma

Lipoma of the large bowel is a rare, benign, often single, and submucosal adipose-tissue tumor. Occasionally, lipomas may present as multiple yellowish polyps. Lipoma is seen in adults and affects both genders. Large lipomas can cause constipation, abdominal pain, rectal bleeding, and intussusception.

Histopathology Lipoma is an encapsulated mass composed of mature adipose tissue exhibiting small, uniform nuclei. Focal fat necrosis may be seen.

Immuno-Profile Lipomas are immunoreactive for vimentin and S-100 protein.

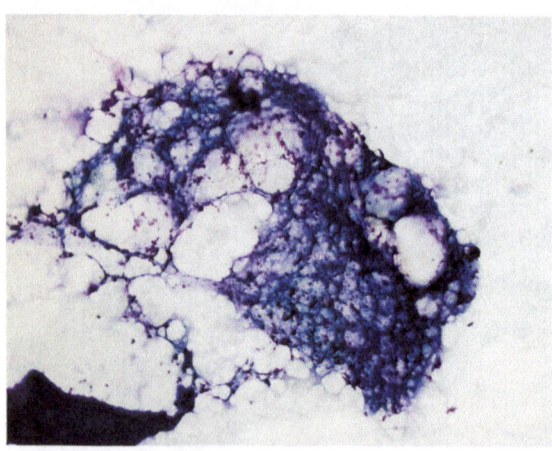

FIG. 6.3. Lipoma. ERUS-FNA shows a fragment of mature adipose tissue with large single vacuoles pushing the small nuclei to the periphery (DiffQuik stain, X200).

Molecular Profile One half of lipomas show aberrations in the chromosome 12q13–15 segment. The target gene for rearrangement is *HMGA2* (HMGA2/LLP and HMGA2/RDC1).

FNA Findings Aspirated smears show small fragments of mature adipocytes and grossly visible fat vacuoles (Fig. 6.3). The adipocytes contain a large, single lipid vacuole and a small nucleus located at the periphery.

ERUS Features Lipoma is a well-defined, often hyperechogenic submucosal mass (Figs. 6.4 and 6.5).

Schwannoma

Schwannoma is a rare, benign colorectal tumor of adults and affects both genders equally. The tumor is usually a well-circumscribed submucosal mass.

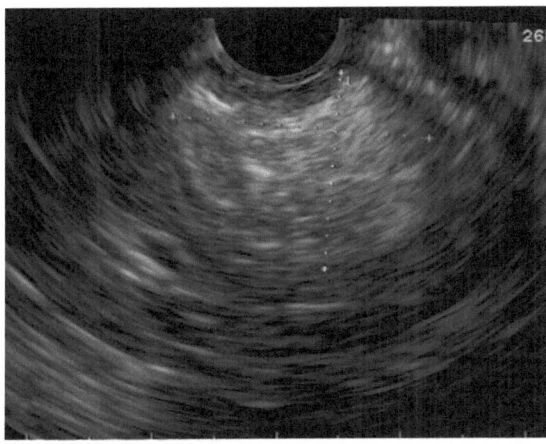

Fɪɢ. 6.4. Lipoma. Linear EUS showing a large iso- and hyperechoic pedunculated polypoid mass that probably originated from the submucosal layer (calipers). The muscularis propria is intact (hypoechoic band inferior to the lower caliper). Retrosigmoid resection revealed a 3.5 cm submucosal lipoma. (Courtesy of Drs. Vikesh K. Singh and Joanna Law, The Johns Hopkins Hospital, Maryland, USA).

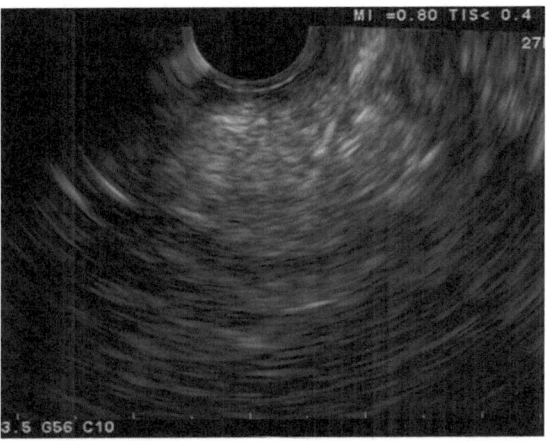

Fɪɢ. 6.5. ERUS-FNA of a submucosal mass, with the sampling needle inside the mass. (Courtesy of Drs. Vikesh K. Singh and Joanna Law, The Johns Hopkins Hospital, Maryland, USA).

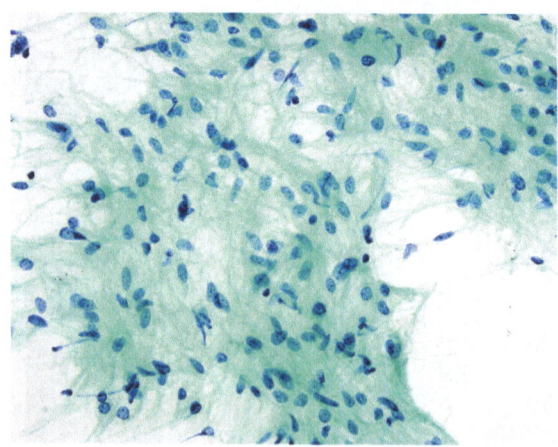

Fig. 6.6. Schwannoma. Loosely cohesive tissue fragment with irregular borders. Round to oval to spindle-shaped nuclei with tapered or pointed ends embedded in a fibrillary stroma. Notice the sprinkled small lymphocytes (Papanicolaou stain, X400).

Histopathology Schwannoma is unencapsulated and is surrounded by lymphocytes. Intralesional lymphocytes can also be seen. The tumor pattern is spindle- or plexiform. The spindle cells are arranged in interlacing bundles; however, in contrast with peripheral Schwannomas or GISTs, a distinct palisading is not identified. The plexiform pattern shows nodules of spindle cells. Focal nuclear atypia or rare mitotic figures are occasionally seen.

Immuno-Profile The cells are immunoreactive for S-100 protein and GFAP and nonreactive for c-Kit, smooth-muscle actin, and desmin; CD34 immunoreactivity may be focal and weak.

Molecular Profile Gastrointestinal Schwannomas are not associated with c-Kit or with neurofibromatosis 2 (*NF2*) gene mutations.

FNA Findings On cytology, the smear shows spindle cells arranged singly or in tissue fragments. The nuclei are oval or wavy. Scattered small lymphocytes, an important clue for the diagnosis, are always present and must be thoroughly searched (Fig. 6.6).

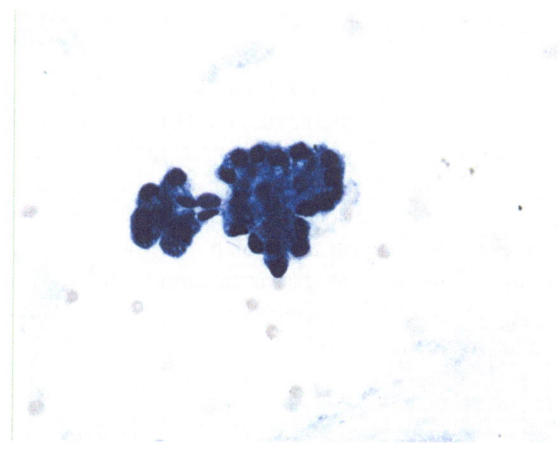

Fɪɢ. 6.7.   Benign acinar cells with uniform round, eccentrically placed nuclei and granular cytoplasm in an ectopic pancreas (DiffQuik stain, X400. Courtesy of Dr. Yener Erozan, The Johns Hopkins Hospital, Maryland, USA).

ERUS Features   The mass is relatively well-defined, hypoechogenic, and submucosal. Features are indistinguishable from those of GIST.

Heterotopic Pancreas

Ectopic pancreatic tissue is a relatively frequent congenital anomaly. It is most common in the upper gastrointestinal tract, including the stomach, duodenum, and jejunum, and less common in the lower GI tract, particularly the colon.

Gross examination reveals a well-circumscribed, lobulated, yellow tan, firm nodule. Central umbilication is seen in cases located in the submucosa. Histologic examination shows normal pancreatic acini and ducts. Islet cells are seen in less than half of the cases. Ectopic pancreas is immunoreactive for amylase, lipase, and trypsinogen. No genetic abnormality is detected. Cytology smears show clusters of benign pancreatic acini and ductal epithelium (Fig. 6.7).

Gastric Heterotopia

Gastric heterotopia is a rare condition that may occur in the anus and rectum. It is slightly more common in males than in females, with a mean age of 21 years. Patients complain of rectal pain, bleeding, or irritable bowel syndrome. In asymptomatic patients gastric heterotopia can be identified incidentally on cancer screening. The lesion may appear as a polyp, diverticulum, or ulcer on colonoscopy. A fundic type gastric mucosa is the most common histologic finding. Cytology smears show benign columnar, parietal, and oxyntic cells.

ERUS-FNA of Malignant Intramural Colorectal Masses

Colorectal Adenocarcinoma

Colorectal carcinoma is the most common carcinoma of the gastrointestinal tract. It is the third most common cancer in the United States, affecting males and females equally at a mean age of 60 years. It is the second leading cancer-related cause of death. The pathogenesis of colorectal carcinoma is related to personal, familial, and environmental risk factors. Individuals with a history of inflammatory bowel disease (ulcerative colitis, Crohn's disease), adenomas (tubular, villous, or tubulovillous), sessile serrated polyps, prior colorectal cancer, and/or those who have a first-degree relative with invasive colorectal cancer are at high risk of developing colorectal cancer. Inherited syndromes, such as Lynch syndrome (also known as hereditary nonpolyposis colorectal cancer), polyposis syndromes including classical familial adenomatous polyposis, attenuated familial adenomatous polyposis, *MUTYH*-associated polyposis (MAP), juvenile polyposis syndrome, Peutz-Jeghers syndrome, serrated polyposis syndrome, Cowden syndrome, and Li-Fraumeni syndrome also are associated with a high risk of colorectal cancer. Diets high in red meat or processed meat and low in fiber, as well as smoking, alcohol consumption, a high body mass index, and a low level of physical activity are considered personal lifestyle risk factors. Colorectal cancer screening, recommended at age of 50 for men and women with average risk, has decreased the mortality rate due to colorectal cancer because of early detection of precancerous lesions. Colorectal cancer most commonly occurs in the cecum, ascending colon, sigmoid colon, and rarely in the anal canal (where it must be distinguished from extension from a rectal primary). The tumor is either exophytic or infiltrating.

Histopathology The well- to moderately-differentiated colorectal carcinoma consists of elongated, pseudostratified columnar cells forming glands of various sizes. The cells exhibit a high nuclear-to-cytoplasmic ratio, hyperchromatic nuclei with prominent nucleoli, and moderate amounts of finely vacuolated cytoplasm. Variable mitotic activity, foci of necrosis, acute and chronic inflammatory response, and pools of excess mucin are common findings. Tumor invasion promotes a desmoplastic stromal reaction. Poorly differentiated carcinoma grows in solid sheets with no distinct glandular formation. Focal squamous differentiation or neuroendocrine differentiation can be seen. Other histologic variants of colorectal carcinoma are mucinous, signet-ring-cell, and, less commonly, clear cell, anaplastic, hepatoid, basaloid (cloacogenic), and medullary.

Immuno-Profile Colorectal adenocarcinoma is immunoreactive for CK20, CDX2, CEA, MUC1, and MUC3. CK7 is negative; however, it can be expressed in rectal adenocarcinoma. The tumor cells are nonimmunoreactive with DPC4 (SMAD4), HepPar1, and MUC2.

Molecular Profile RAS mutations including both *KRAS* and *NRAS* should be investigated in all patients who have metastatic colorectal adenocarcinoma; at the very least, exon 2 *KRAS* mutation status should be determined. *KRAS* and *NRAS* mutations are similar in both primary and/or metastatic colorectal adenocarcinoma. *BRAF* V600E mutation is associated with a poor prognosis. Testing for *NRAS*, *KRAS*, and *BRAF* V600E mutations is performed on formalin-fixed, paraffin-embedded tissue; PCR-based amplification and DNA sequencing are the recommended methods. Microsatellite

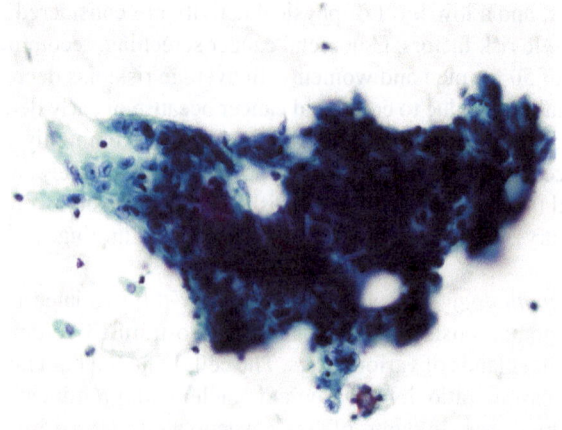

FIG. 6.8. Rectal adenocarcinoma. The smear shows a complex flat aggre-
gate of malignant cells with large nuclei, irregular nuclear membranes, and
prominent nucleoli. Pseudo-glandular lumens are present (Papanicolaou
stain, X400).

instability is associated mainly with mucinous adenocarcinoma or
poorly differentiated carcinoma.

FNA Findings The cytomorphologic findings are similar to the
histologic findings. The malignant cells are arranged as single or
in clusters or as tissue fragments. Glandular or acinar formation
is seen in well- or moderately-differentiated adenocarcinoma. The
cells are tall and columnar, with a high nuclear-to-cytoplasmic ratio. The nuclei are elongated and hyperchromatic, with prominent
nucleoli and atypical mitotic figures. The cells contain moderate
and finely vacuolar cytoplasm. Necrosis and inflammatory cells are
commonly prominent in the background (Fig. 6.8).

ERUS Features The mass is heterogeneous and hypoechoic, originates in the mucosa, and shows variable invasion into the wall, with
irregular infiltrating margins. ERUS accurately shows the depth of
tumor invasion (Fig. 6.9) and evaluates regional lymph nodes, if
they are larger than 2–3 mm. It is difficult to evaluate the primary
site of the tumor in the mucosal layer when the tumor is ulcerated.

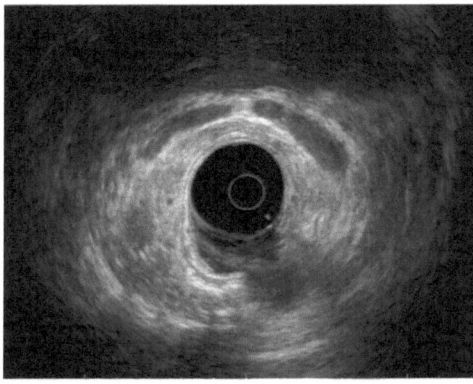

Fig. 6.9. Rectal adenocarcinoma. Transrectal radial EUS shows tumor invasion through the submucosa (arrow) into deep layers. (Courtesy of Drs. Vikesh K. Singh and Joanna Law, The Johns Hopkins Hospital, Maryland, USA).

Squamous Cell Carcinoma

Primary colonic squamous carcinoma is exceedingly rare. Risk factors include mechanical trauma, local radiotherapy, and chronic schistosomiasis. In the absence of risk factors or a history of a distant squamous primary, colonic squamous carcinoma is a diagnosis of exclusion. Squamous cell carcinoma of the anus (15% of anal cancers) and the anal canal (80% of anal cancers) is seen in adults and mainly affects females in the sixth and seventh decades of life. In the last 20 years, there has been a shift in the age of diagnosis, with a higher incidence in younger individuals, more commonly in those with immunosuppression, particularly HIV. Rectal bleeding, a nodular or ulcerated mass, and pain are common clinical findings. The tumor can invade deeply in perirectal soft tissue, both proximally and distally. The treatment of choice includes combined neoadjuvant chemoradiation therapy, which achieves a remarkably good response, followed by radical surgery (abdominoperineal resection) only for persistent or locally recurrent tumors.

Histopathology The tumors vary in their differentiation, keratinization, and subtypes. Keratinized squamous cell carcinoma is characterized by intercellular bridges and keratin pearls. Large-cell, non-keratinizing squamous cell carcinoma lacks keratin pearls and may present diagnostic challenges. Subtypes of squamous cell carcinoma include verrucous carcinoma, carcinoma with mucinous microcysts (mucoepidermoid), and small-cell (anaplastic) carcinoma, the latter two with a poor prognosis. Immunostains differentiate small-cell anaplastic carcinoma from small-cell undifferentiated neuroendocrine carcinoma.

Immuno-Profile Squamous cell carcinoma is immunoreactive for P40, P63, and CK5/6. High-risk human papilloma viruses (HPV) are detected in most squamous cell carcinomas of the anus and anal canal. HPV-related squamous cell carcinoma is immunoreactive for the HPV surrogate marker P16.

Molecular Profile Squamous cell carcinoma of the anus shows a low rate of epidermal growth factor receptor (*EGFR*) and *KRAS* mutations and a high surface expression of EGFR, findings similar to those found in squamous carcinomas of the head and neck. HPV DNA genotypes 16 and 18 can be detected by PCR. The *c-myc* amplification is detected in one-third of anal squamous cell carcinomas. Gains and losses in various chromosomes have been detected by genomic hybridization.

FNA Findings Cytology smears of keratinizing squamous cell carcinoma show variably pleomorphic cells with bizarre shapes, orangeophilic cytoplasm, and hyperchromatic nuclei; necrosis and tumor diathesis can be seen in the background (Fig. 6.10). Non-keratinizing squamous cell carcinoma is characterized by relatively uniform malignant cells arranged in sheets or individually showing dense cytoplasm, hyperchromatic nuclei with irregular chromatin distribution, and one or more nucleoli. Histomorphology and judicious use of immunostains can be performed on cell-block slides (Fig. 6.11).

ERUS Features The findings are similar to those described for colorectal adenocarcinoma (Figs. 6.12, 6.13, 6.14).

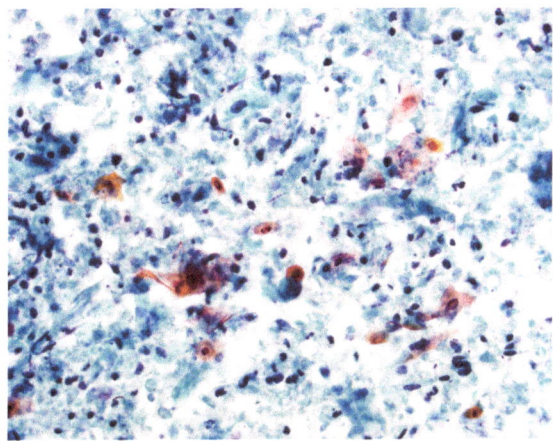

FIG. 6.10. Keratinizing squamous cell carcinoma shows scattered single, atypical orangeophilic squamous cells in a background of necrosis (Papanicolaou stain, X400).

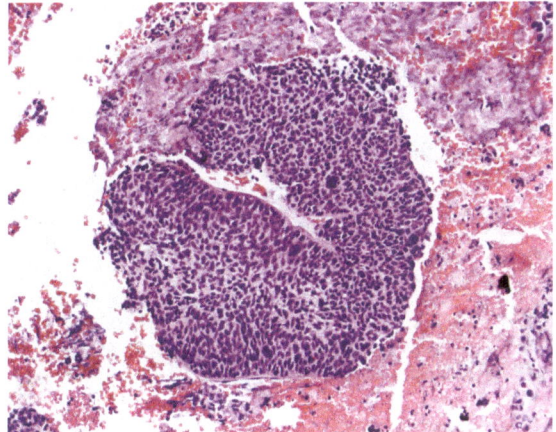

FIG. 6.11. Fragments of squamous cell carcinoma with basaloid features in a background of necrosis in a cell-block preparation (H&E, X200).

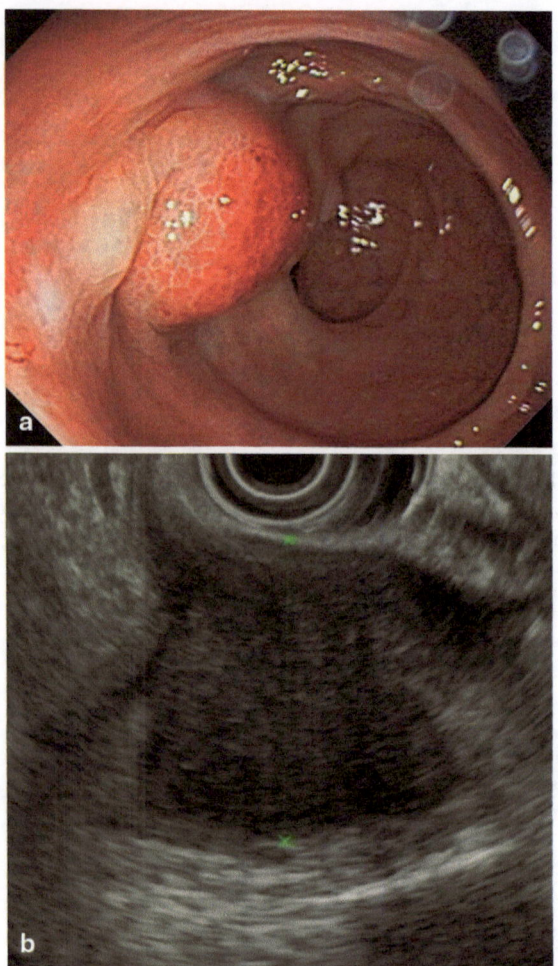

FIG. 6.12. **a**, **b** Rectosigmoidoscopy demonstrates a large polyp with an erythematous overlying mucosa in a patient with basaloid squamous cell carcinoma of the rectum (**a**). Linear EUS shows a 3.5 cm hypoechoic, irregular mass extending through the mucosa and muscularis mucosa (**b**). (Courtesy of Drs. Vikesh K. Singh and Joanna Law, The Johns Hopkins Hospital, Maryland, USA).

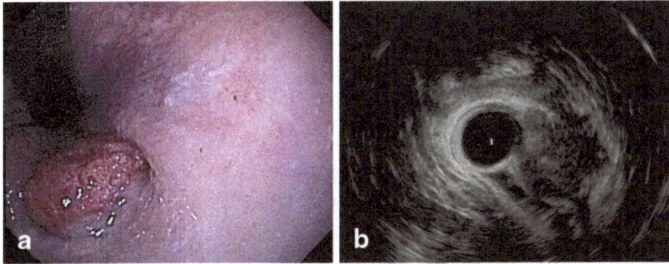

FIG. 6.13. **a, b** Flexible sigmoidoscopy shows a polypoid, fungating mass, seen on retroreflexed view in a patient with rectal squamous cell carcinoma in situ (**a**). On radial EUS imaging, there is an ill-defined hypoechoic mass breaching the muscularis propria (**b**). (Courtesy of Drs. Vikesh K. Singh and Joanna Law, The Johns Hopkins Hospital, Maryland, USA).

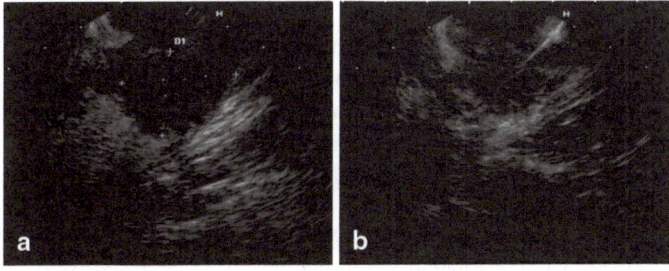

FIG. 6.14. **a, b** On linear EUS imaging, this superficial anal lesion spares the muscularis propria and does not involve any sphincters (**a**). A linear echoendoscope image shows the superficial anal lesion sparing the muscularis propria at the time of undergoing EUS-guided FNA (**b**). (Courtesy of Drs. Vikesh K. Singh and Joanna Law, The Johns Hopkins Hospital, Maryland, USA).

Malignant Melanoma

Primary malignant melanoma of the anorectum (the most common site of the GI tract) is very rare (<1% of colorectal malignant tumors) and is associated with a poor prognosis. Anorectal melanoma is a polypoid or fungating intraluminal tumor which appears black if it contains melanin pigments and can be mistaken clinically for anal tags or hemorrhoids. Lesions often originate in the anorectal transition zone, where melanocytes are found. One-third of melanomas are amelanotic. The prognosis is poor, with a 5-year survival rate of <20%.

Histopathology The *in situ* component, junctional nests, pagetoid spread, and satellite lesions are often found, confirming the anorectal origin; however, ulcerated lesions may lack these features. The tumor exhibits epithelioid, spindle, lymphocyte-like, or mixed cell patterns. Epithelioid melanocytes show abundant eosinophilic cytoplasm and nuclei with prominent nucleoli. Pigmented melanoma shows brown–black granular or fine dusty cytoplasmic pigment that is also found in melanophages. Nuclear intracytoplasmic inclusions, nuclear grooves, nuclear polymorphism, atypical mitosis, and necrosis are other features found in melanoma.

Immuno-Profile Anorectal melanoma is immunoreactive for S-100 protein, HMB45, Melan-A/Mart1, tyrosinase, microphthalmia transcription factor (MITF), nestin, and SOX2. CD117 (c-Kit) is positive in >80% of anorectal melanomas. The tumor is nonreactive for smooth-muscle actin, CD34, and AE1/AE3.

Molecular Profile *BRAF*, *KIT*, *NRAS*, and *PIK3CA* are the most common genes evaluated for mutation. *BRAF* mutation is found in <5% and *c-kit*-activating mutations are seen in 20% of anorectal melanomas and do not correlate with CD117 expression. It should be emphasized that *c-kit* mutations must be evaluated in all colorectal primary and metastatic melanomas, because their identification is associated with an excellent response to therapy with tyrosine kinase inhibitors.

FNA Findings Smears show numerous malignant single cells. The cells are round, oval, plasmacytoid, or spindled. Anisocytosis is seen in most cases. Giant malignant cells are occasionally seen. The nuclear-to-cytoplasmic ratio is increased. Prominent nucleoli, binucleation, and intranuclear pseudoinclusions are other common features. Malignant cells with intracytoplasmic melanin or pigmented macrophages are helpful diagnostic features (Fig. 6.15).

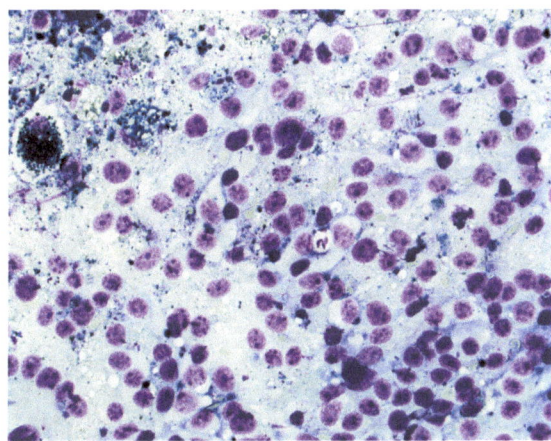

FIG. 6.15. Malignant melanoma. Numerous plasmacytoid malignant cells with prominent nucleoli and scattered melanophages with cytoplasmic pigment are seen (DiffQuik Stain, X400).

The differential diagnosis includes, but is not limited to poorly differentiated carcinoma, signet-ring cell carcinoma, spindle cell tumors including high-risk GIST (CD34 and DOG-1 are positive), and leiomyosarcoma, lymphoma, and small-cell carcinoma.

ERUS Features The tumor may involve all layers of the rectal wall. Depending upon the depth of invasion, the ERUS image exhibits an ill-defined hypoechoic mass with irregular margins, penetrating the submucosa and deeper layers.

Lymphoma

Colorectal lymphoma is very uncommon, representing 6–20 % of GI lymphomas. Rectal lymphoma, either as a primary (less than 0.5 %) or as a manifestation of a systemic disseminated disease, is even rarer. Colorectal lymphomas are seen mostly in males in their sixth to seventh decades of life. Inflammatory bowel disease and a compromised immune system are considered risk factors. Abdom-

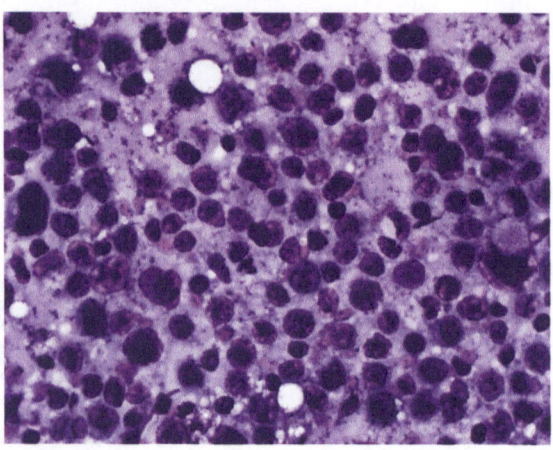

FIG. 6.16. Diffuse large B-cell lymphoma with markedly atypical en-larged lymphocytes. The nuclei exhibit an irregular and thickened nuclear membrane (DiffQuik Stain, X400).

inal pain is the chief complaint. Most colorectal lymphomas are of the B-cell type in Western countries. Diffuse large B-cell lym-phoma (Fig. 6.16) and lymphoma arising from mucosa-associated lymphoid tissue (MALT) are the most common types. T cell lym-phomas have a high incidence in Asia.

Colorectal lymphomas manifest as polypoid masses and, less commonly, as diffuse mucosal nodules, or circumferential lesions causing concentric thickening of the wall. The surface mucosa can be normal or ulcerated. The circumferential lesions, even if large, do not cause luminal obstruction.

Histopathology Microscopic examination is significant for infiltra-tion of a monotonous population of lymphocytes, and the morphol-ogy depends upon the type of lymphoma.

Immuno-Profile CD20 and CD3 are two main immunostains for detecting B-cell and T-cell lymphocytes, respectively. CD10, bcl-2, and bcl-6 are seen in follicular lymphomas. Flow cytometry is paramount for making the diagnosis in FNA samples.

Molecular Profile Cytogenetic studies are widely used in lymphomas. For example, diffuse large B-cell lymphoma and follicular-cell lymphomas are associated with t(14:18) and t(3:14); MALT lymphoma shows trisomy 3 and 18 and t(1:14) and t(11:18).

FNA Findings The cytomorphology of lymphomas varies for the different subtypes. Aspirated material is submitted for flow cytometry studies following on-site immediate interpretation.

ERUS Features Hypoechoic masses with irregular borders are present. Regional lymph nodes involved by lymphoma are round and well-circumscribed with sharp margins, and deeply hypoechoic ("pseudocystic" appearance).

Leiomyosarcoma

Colorectal leiomyosarcoma, a malignant neoplasm of smooth-muscle origin, is slightly more common in men than in women, with a mean age of 58 years. Grossly, it may appear as mainly a polypoid intraluminal mass, or occasionally as a plaque-like lesion with transmural growth. Mucosal ulceration is common. The tumor is firm and gray-white to tan on sectioning.

Histopathology Microscopically, the tumor consists of spindle cells with oval to mildly elongated nuclei and eosinophilic cytoplasm. Nuclear pleomorphism, high mitotic activity, and focal necrosis are also seen.

Immuno-Profile Leiomyosarcoma is reactive with α-SMA in almost all cases, and with desmin in close to half of the cases, and is negative for CD34, CD117 (c-kit), and S-100 protein.

Molecular Profile In contrast to GIST, leiomyosarcoma shows no *c-kit*-activating mutations.

FNA Findings Smears show malignant spindle cells arranged singly or in large tissue fragments. The nuclei are hyperchromatic

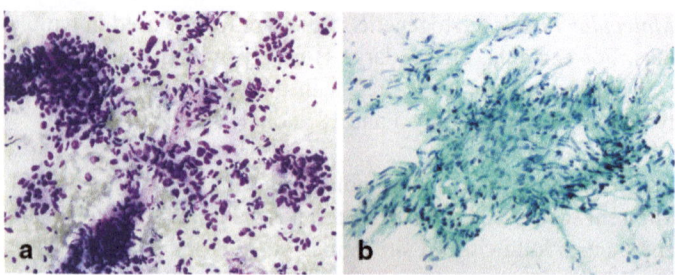

F<small>IG</small>. 6.17. **a, b** Leiomyosarcoma characterized by spindle cells of vari-able sizes and shapes, arranged singly and in clusters embedded in a scant fibrillary stroma (**a, b**). Cytomorphology is similar to that of GIST; dif-ferentiation between the two by means of immunostains and or molecular tests must be done because of its therapeutic and prognostic implications. (**a**, DiffQuik Stain, X400; **b**, Papanicolaou stain, X400).

and elongated, with blunted ends. The cytoplasm is abundant and dense. Naked nuclei, mitoses, nuclear pleomorphism, anisonucleo-sis, multinucleation, and necrosis are other common features found in high-grade leiomyosarcoma (Fig. 6.17a, b).

ERUS Features Examination shows a well-defined, hypoechoic, intramural polypoid mass. High-grade tumors show irregular tu-mor margins and a heterogeneous echotexture.

Metastases

Metastatic tumors may present as a submucosal or perirectal mass, or an enlarged lymph node. Distant primary sites include, but are not limited to the stomach, breast, gallbladder, pancreas, kidney, or lung. Gastric carcinoma may invade the rectal mucosa in a diffuse pattern identical to that seen in linitis plastica of the primary site. Metastatic urothelial, prostatic, and squamous cell carcinomas of the female genital tract, including the vagina, vulva, and uterine cervix, are examples of sources in nearby organs. Metastatic ma-lignant melanoma from skin, eye, and anus is seen more commonly than metastasis from primary melanoma of the rectum.

ERUS-FNA of Intramural Colorectal Tumors of Uncertain Behavior

Neuroendocrine Neoplasms

Neuroendocrine neoplasms (NENs) can occur in any part of the large bowel, including the colon, rectum, and anal canal. The mean age at the time of diagnosis is 58 years, and it mainly affects males (M:F ratio 3:1).

The spectrum of clinicopathologic features of NENs ranges from low grade (carcinoid tumor, grade 1), to intermediate grade (grade 2), to high grade (small- and large-cell neuroendocrine carcinoma, grade 3). Carcinoids are common in the rectum and NE carcinomas in the colon, especially the right colon.

Rectal carcinoid tumors are more common than are colonic carcinoids. Rectal carcinoids tend to be small, flat, or polypoid and can be resected endoscopically; regional or distant lymph node metastases may be seen at the time of diagnosis. Cross section of the formalin-fixed carcinoid tumor shows a characteristic yellow appearance. Unlike gastric and small-bowel carcinoid tumors, which are present with carcinoid syndrome in up to 50 % of cases, colorectal carcinoid is rarely associated with carcinoid syndrome that includes diarrhea and elevated urinary 5-hydroxyindoleacetic acid).

Colonic NE carcinomas have a larger size, a poorer prognosis, a higher rate of undifferentiated histology, and a more aggressive clinical behavior among all gastrointestinal NE carcinomas. Large-cell NE carcinoma is the most common, followed by small-cell carcinoma and mixed carcinoma.

Histopathology Carcinoid tumors show islands, ribbons, sheets, glands, and trabecular arrangements. Rectal carcinoids have the characteristic trabecular pattern, whereas trabecular, nodular, or mixed pattern is seen mostly in colonic carcinoids. The cells are relatively small and uniform, with centrally located round to oval nuclei surrounded by a scant to moderate amount of finely granular cytoplasm. Pleomorphism, mitoses, and necrosis are minimal; however, these features are prominent in NE carcinomas.

Immuno-Profile Carcinoid tumors are immunoreactive for broad-spectrum cytokeratins (AE1/AE3) and neuroendocrine markers including synaptophysin, chromogranin, CD56, neuron-specific enolase, and Leu 7 (CD57). Chromogranin stain is strong and diffuse in carcinoids, and focal or negative in NE carcinomas; synaptophysin is positive in poorly differentiated NE carcinomas. Ki-67 is low and reflects the low proliferation index of the tumor.

Molecular Profile NENs of the transverse colon to the rectum express transforming growth factor α (TGF-α) and EGFR. Overexpression of the *p16* and *p53* genes is observed in the majority of NENs of the GI tract. Components of the retinoblastoma (*RB*) gene pathway such as RB protein (pRB), $p16^{INK4a}$, and cyclin D1 have been found to be variably altered in NENs of the GI tract; the loss of pRB may be a predictor of metastases in rectal carcinoids.

FNA Findings Cytology smears of carcinoid tumors show high cellularity, loosely cohesive cell groups, and single, small, uniform cells with centrally located nuclei and a moderate amount of granular cytoplasm. The stippled nuclei display granular, unevenly distributed chromatin (Fig. 6.18). Higher degrees of necrosis, cellular pleomorphism, and nucleolar prominence are more evident in higher-grade NE carcinomas.

ERUS Features Examination shows a well-circumscribed polypoid, hypoechoic, homogeneous, and well-circumscribed mass localized in the submucosal layer of the colorectal wall. Occasionally, the tumor may involve superficial and deep layers. Poorly differentiated NE carcinomas have a large size, infiltrating margins, and a heterogeneous echotexture similar to that of other high-grade malignancies.

Gastrointestinal Stromal Tumor

GIST of the large bowel occurs mostly in adults older than 50 years and is mostly malignant. Colonic GISTs are more common than leiomyosarcomas and are typically transmural, with both intraluminal and outward-bulging components.

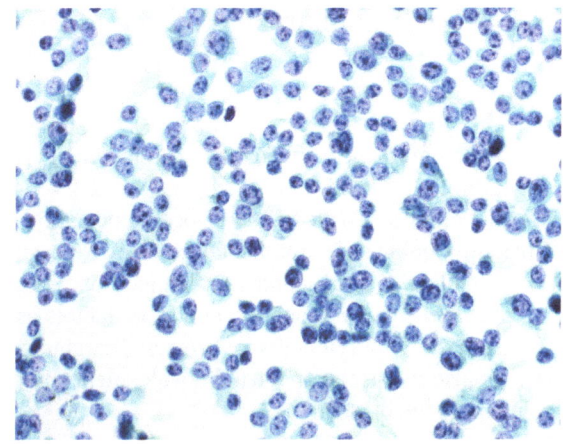

FIG. 6.18. Carcinoid tumor. Smears show relatively small cells with round to oval nuclei and a moderate amount of cytoplasm. The chromatin is stippled, and the nucleus is located eccentrically (Papanicolaou stain, X400).

The histopathology, immune-profile, molecular profile, and cytomorphology of colorectal GISTs are similar to those of GISTs of the upper GI tract and have been described in Chap. 5. Briefly, spindle cell GISTs are more common than epithelioid GISTs; they are reactive with CD117 (c-kit), DOG-1, and CD34 immunostains. *C-Kit* gene mutation is seen in most cases. The differential diagnosis includes, but is not limited to Schwannoma and smooth-muscle tumors. Of note, colorectal GIST is more aggressive than leiomyosarcoma; thus, an accurate distinction between the two, by use of immunostains and molecular tests if needed, is paramount.

ERUS shows a well-circumscribed mass arising in the fourth layer (muscularis propria) of the GI wall. The mass is hypoechoic, round to oval, and has a homogeneous echotexture. A size larger than 5 cm, hyperechoic foci, cystic change, and irregular margins are sonographic features consistent with a high-risk GIST.

ERUS-FNA of Extramural Colorectal Masses

Urothelial Carcinoma

Urothelial carcinoma is the most common carcinoma of the urinary bladder. Males are affected more than females and whites more than African Americans, with an age of occurrence at 50 years or more. Cigarette smoking, environmental exposure to certain chemicals such as aniline dyes containing arylamines, and medications including phenacetin and cyclophosphamide are factors associated with increased risk for development of urothelial carcinoma. Schistosomiasis is also a risk factor for the development of squamous cell carcinoma of the bladder.

Histopathology Urothelial carcinoma shows solid nests and cords surrounded by reactive desmoplastic stroma. Pleomorphic bizarre cells, occasionally multinucleated, are seen. Focal glandular and/or squamous differentiation may be noted in high-grade carcinomas.

Immuno-Profile Urothelial carcinoma is immunoreactive for GATA3, CK7, CK20, B-catenin, thrombomodulin, and uroplakin.

Molecular Profile The cyclin-dependent kinase inhibitor 2 A (*CD-KN2A*) gene is frequently deleted in bladder carcinoma. Fibroblast growth factor receptor 3 and the *RAS* genes are mutated in most nonmuscle-invasive urothelial carcinomas.

FNA Findings Smears show large pleomorphic malignant cells with a high nuclear-to-cytoplasmic ratio and a plasmacytoid appearance. The nuclei are hyperchromatic, with coarse chromatin and irregular nuclear borders. Atypical mitotic figures and degenerative changes can be seen. The cytoplasm is scant to moderate and finely vacuolated in most cases (Fig. 6.19a). "Cercariform" cells, when present, are useful clues to suggest a primary urothelial carcinoma.

ERUS Features Examination shows an ill-defined mass in the perirectal area infiltrating the muscularis propria toward the mucosa layer, or a perirectal lymph node with features suspicious of metastasis (Fig. 6.19b).

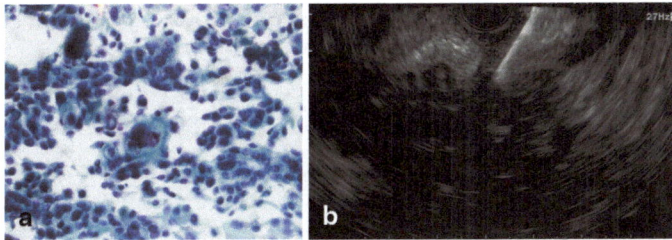

Fig. 6.19. **a, b** Urothelial carcinoma. Hypercellular smear showing cells with moderate pleomorphism. Note the extremely large cells in the center (**a**). "Cercariform" cells were also found in the smears (**a**, Papanicolaou stain, X400). The transrectal linear EUS image shows an ill-defined irregular mass, undergoing EUS-guided FNA (**b**). (**b**, Courtesy of Drs. Vikesh K. Singh and Joanna Law, The Johns Hopkins Hospital, Maryland, USA).

Prostatic Adenocarcinoma

Prostatic adenocarcinoma is the most common cancer, and the second most common cause of cancer-related deaths, in males. Twenty percent of men in the USA are diagnosed with prostate cancer during their lifetime, more common in males of 50 years of age or older. Patients remain asymptomatic in most instances, but occasionally may have back pain due to carcinoma metastatic to the lumbar spine. Prostate specific antigen (PSA), although non-specific, is elevated in most cases.

Histopathology Acinar or conventional adenocarcinoma comprises the majority of prostatic carcinomas. Mucinous, endometrial, signet-ring-cell, small cell, basaloid, prostatic duct, and carcinosarcomas are other types of prostate carcinomas. The cellular arrangement of the tumor is related to the degree of tumor differentiation. Acinar adenocarcinoma exhibits cuboidal to columnar epithelial cells with abundant cytoplasm, enlarged nuclei, and prominent nucleoli.

Immuno-Profile Prostatic adenocarcinoma is immunoreactive with PSA, P501s, NKX3, and PSMA. Both urothelial and prostatic adenocarcinomas are immunoreactive with SNF5. High-grade

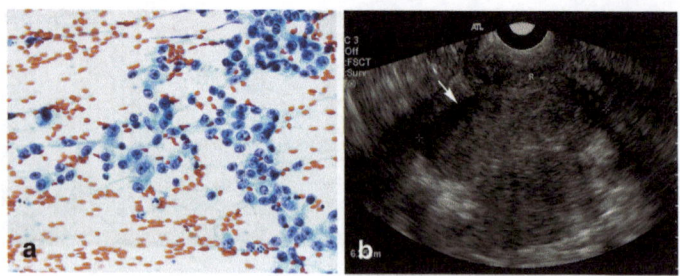

FIG. 6.20. **a, b** Prostatic adenocarcinoma with cells arranged singly or loosely cohesive, forming glands (*right upper portion*). The nuclei contain prominent nucleoli, and the cytoplasm is delicate and finely vacuolated (**a**, Papanicolaou stain, X400). On transrectal ultrasound, the transverse plane shows a large solid mass (*white arrow*) anterior to the rectum ®. (**b**, Courtesy of Dr. Sheila Sheth, The Johns Hopkins Hospital, Maryland, USA).

prostatic adenocarcinoma may lose immunoreactivity to most prostatic adenocarcinoma markers and may show neuroendocrine immunoreactivity with synaptophysin, chromogranin, and CD56, and may have a high proliferation index (Ki-56) similar to that of small cell carcinoma.

Molecular Profile Missense mutation (G84E, rs138213197) in the gene homeobox B13 (*HOXB13*) has been associated with an increased risk of hereditary prostate cancer.

FNA Findings The smears are usually cellular and show tissue fragments, loose cell clusters, microacini, and single cells. The cells are large, with abundant finely vacuolated cytoplasm, large nuclei, and prominent nucleoli. Nuclei are hyperchromatic with thick, irregular nuclear membranes, and one or two prominent nucleoli (Fig. 6.20a). Microacinar formation and nuclear features are useful clues for the diagnosis of metastatic prostate cancer. High-grade prostatic adenocarcinomas may exhibit neuroendocrine features.

ERUS Features Prostatic adenocarcinoma can be detected on ERUS either as metastatic carcinoma involving perirectal lymph nodes, or locally invading the rectum, presenting as a submucosal intramural nodule/mass with an intact mucosa (Fig. 6.20b).

Female Genital Tract

Endometriosis Endometriosis affects the GI tract, mainly the sigmoid colon, in up to 37% of patients who have pelvic endometriosis. Clinically, colorectal endometriosis can mimic inflammatory bowel disease, ischemic colitis, or even colorectal neoplasms. Endometriosis can induce secondary smooth-muscle hypertrophy and result in bowel obstruction. The overlying mucosa may show ulcerative and inflammatory changes or small areas of hemorrhage.

Histopathology Endometriosis involves the serosa and muscularis propria, inducing a fibroblastic response and serosal adhesions. Endometrial glands surrounded by endometrial stroma, as well as hemosiderin-laden macrophages, are present along with fibrosis and hypertrophic smooth muscle.

Immuno-Profile The endometrial glands are immunoreactive for ER and PR. The stromal cells are immunoreative for CD10 in addition to ER and PR. CD68 and iron stain can highlight the hemosiderin-laden macrophages. CEA and CDX2 immunostains are negative and differentiate endometriosis from colorectal glandular epithelium.

Molecular Profile A study showed that 16-bp duplication polymorphism in *TP53* (a tumor suppressor gene encoding P53 nuclear phosphorylation) contributes significantly to endometriosis susceptibility in the Mexican population. Micro-RNA-126 may also play a role in the initial development of endometriosis.

FNA Findings The diagnosis of endometriosis by FNA can be made safely if smears show an endometrial-type glandular epithelium, endometrial stroma, and hemosiderin-laden macrophages, particularly in cell-block preparations. However; in most cases one or two of these elements is present, and the diagnosis can be backed up only by a high index of suspicion (Fig. 6.21a, b).

ERUS Features ERUS shows a lesion infiltrating the colorectal wall, mimicking malignancy. ERUS is a valuable tool for detecting

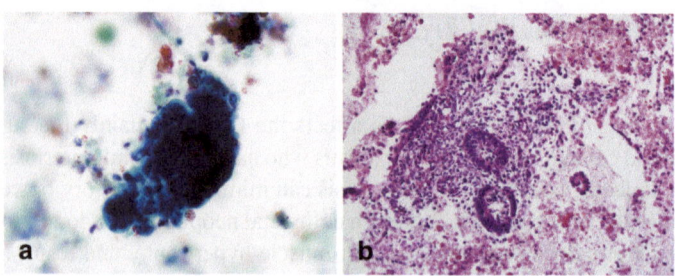

FIG. 6.21. **a, b** Endometriosis. A tissue fragment consists of dense stromal cells in the center, surrounded by cuboidal epithelial cells. The background shows hemosiderin -laden macrophages (out of focus) and debris (**a**). A cell block preparation almost resembling an endometrial biopsy shows both glandular and stromal components (**b**) (A, Papanicolaou stain, X400; B, H&E, X200).

and accurately predicting endometriosis in the muscularis layer; however, it is not as accurate in detecting involvement of the sub-mucosal/mucosal layer. Thus, patient management, bowel resection versus a more conservative approach can not be solely based on ERUS findings.

Malignant Tumors Gynecologic malignant neoplasms include car-cinomas, malignant stromal tumors of the uterus, and carcinosarco-mas. The morphology of these tumors differs based on the primary site of involvement and the tumor cell type. Immunohistochemistry is performed for confirmation of the diagnosis and the primary site. ER, PR, and P53 are positive in carcinomas. CD10 and smooth mus-cle markers (desmin, smooth-muscle actin, muscle-specific actin) are immunoreactive in endometrial stromal sarcoma and in areas with smooth-muscle differentiation, whereas CD117 (c-kit) and H-calde-smon are nonreactive. The tumor cytomorphology in the aspirated material may vary depending upon the tumor type (Fig. 6.22). ERUS shows malignant lesions locally invading the rectal wall and present as a submucosal intramural nodule/mass with an intact mucosal lay-er, or as metastasis to perirectal lymph nodes (Fig. 6.23a, b, c).

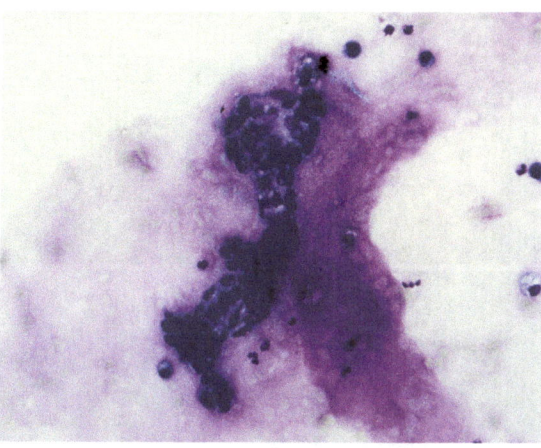

FIG. 6.22. A cystic mass in the peri-rectal space in a patient with ovarian mucinous adenocarcinoma. There is a fragment of epithelial cells with architectural complexity and marked cytologic atypia in a background of abundant mucin and scattered macrophages (DiffQuik stain, X400).

Lymph Nodes

Benign Processes Perirectal lymph nodes may become enlarged due to reactive changes. Histologically, a benign lymph node shows preserved architecture with a mixed T-cell and B-cell population. Flow cytometry shows a mixed polyclonal population of B cells and T cells. Cytology smears shows a polymorphous population of lymphocytes (Fig. 6.24). A reactive lymph node is often oval, hypoechoic, and well-circumscribed (no sharp margins) and has a fatty hilum. As evaluated by Doppler examination, vascularity is limited to the hilum.

Infections and drugs may cause lymphadenopathy. Tuberculosis and fungal infections are common causes of granulomatous inflammation with necrosis; a non-necrotizing granulomatous response is usually seen in sarcoidosis. Granulomatous lymphadenitis may mimic malignancy when evaluated by ultrasound.

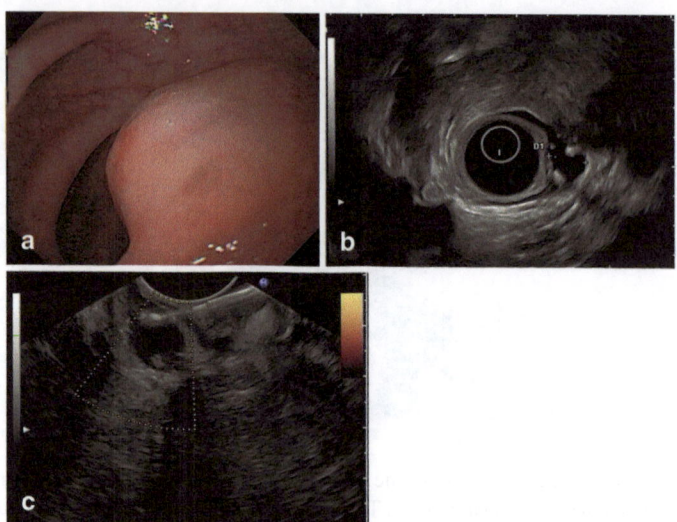

Fig. 6.23. **a–c** A patient with a remote history of ovarian cancer. Flexible sigmoidoscopy shows a subepithelial nodule with intact overlying mucosa (**a**). The radial EUS shows a well-defined anechoic lesion that measures 12.3 mm in maximum diameter (**b**). ERUS-FNA with a linear echoendoscope shows an anechoic cystic mass; the sampling needle is aimed at the mural component of the cyst wall (**c**). Cytology showed a cystic mucinous adenocarcinoma, consistent with the patient's ovarian primary. (**a–c**, Courtesy of Drs. Vikesh K. Singh and Joanna Law, The Johns Hopkins Hospital, Maryland, USA).

Lymphoma Malignant lymphomas are discussed in the section of primary lymphoma of the colorectum. The affected lymph node is enlarged and often has a "pseudocystic," deeply hypoechoic echo-texture with absent fatty hilum; chaotic vascular blood flow is often seen on Doppler examination.

Metastases Perirectal lymph nodes can be enlarged in meta-static malignant neoplasms. Primary tumors include carcinomas, melanoma, and sarcomas and can be regional, in sites such as the rectum, female genital tract, and prostate, or may be distant

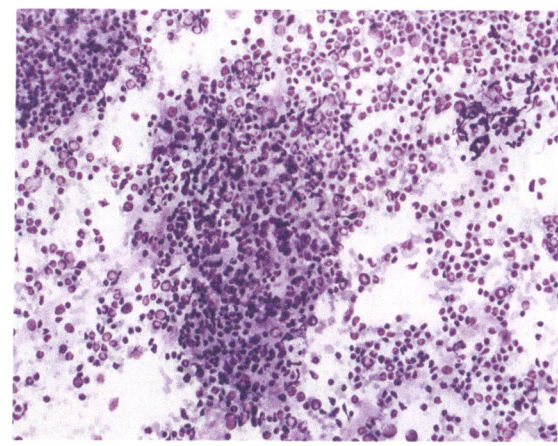

FIG. 6.24. Reactive lymph node. Smears show a polymorphous population of benign reactive lymphoid cells with lymphohistiocytic aggregates (Diffquik stain, X200).

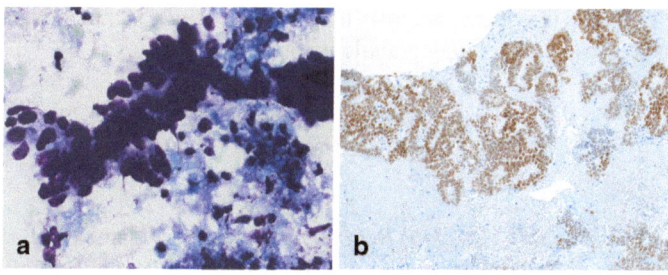

FIG. 6.25. **a, b** Metastatic colorectal adenocarcinoma to a perirectal lymph node. The malignant cells display a disorganized architecture with hyperchromatic elongated nuclei. Necrosis and scattered lymphocytes are seen in the background (**a**). CDX2 immunostain in the cell block highlights the colorectal origin of this carcinoma (**b**) (**a**, DiffQuik stain, X400; **b**, Immunoperoxidase stain, X200).

(Fig. 6.25a). Prior history and immunohistochemistry are helpful for determining the primary site (Fig. 6.25b). ERUS shows a round, deeply hypoechoic, and well-marginated lymph node with absent fatty hilum. Metastatic lymph nodes with irregular margins and a

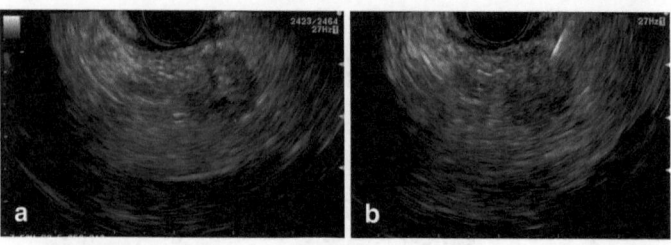

Fɪɢ. 6.26. **a, b** Linear EUS image showing a poorly defined, heterogeneous and hypoechoic node in the perirectal region (**a**). The patient had a history of rectal adenocarcinoma. Linear ERUS shows the malignant lymph node undergoing ERUS- FNA (**b**). (A, B Courtesy of Drs. Vikesh K. Singh and Joanna Law, The Johns Hopkins Hospital, Maryland, USA).

hypoechoic, heterogeneous echotexture indicate necrosis and extracapsular extension (Fig. 6.26a, b). Another helpful clue to the suspicion of metastasis is the identification of an irregular and hypervascular cortex by Doppler examination. It is important to emphasize that cystic necrosis may be seen in metastatic deposits as well as in necrotizing granulomatous processes.

Other Non-tumor Conditions

Developmental Cysts of the Retrorectal Space Developmental cysts are rare congenital anomalies mostly seen in middle-aged women. They are classified as epidermoid, dermoid, tailgut, or neuroenteric cysts.

Epidermoid cyst is unilocular, lined with squamous epithelium without skin adnexae (Fig. 6.27). Dermoid cyst (benign cystic teratoma) is unilocular, lined with squamous epithelium and skin adnexa. Tailgut cysts (retrorectal hamartoma, rectal duplication cyst) are unilocular, lined with colonic, gastric, and/or respiratory epithelium surrounded by smooth muscle, resembling normal mucosa which may communicate with the rectal lumen.

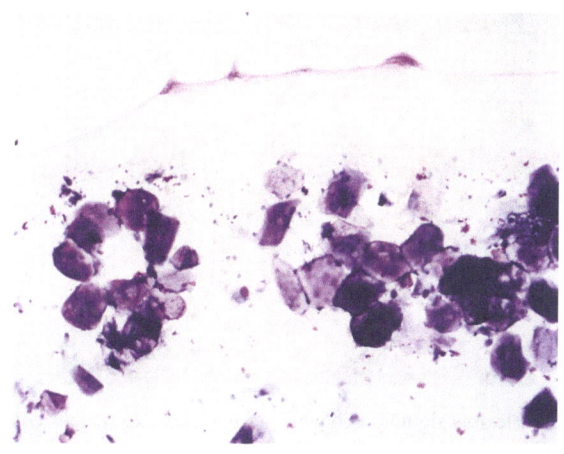

F𝙸𝙶. 6.27. Epidermoid cyst. Smear shows anucleated squamous cells and debris in the background (DiffQuik stain, X200).

FNA is occasionally done when the nature of the cyst is not clear on imaging. Cytologic findings are related to the type of cyst lining epithelium, that is, squamous, columnar ciliated, or glandular cells.

On ERUS, developmental cysts are anechoic and are found in the submucosa. Depending on the type of cyst, sonographically identifiable colorectal layers within the cyst wall may be found.

Fluid Collection Fluid collections, particularly adjacent to the anastomotic site in patients with colorectal cancer resection, and cysts of the genitourinary tract can be investigated by ERUS and ERUS-FNA (Figs. 6.28–6.29a, b). Cytology smears may be acellular in benign conditions.

Perirectal Abscess Abscesses of perirectal or perianal areas are the result of occlusion of anal glands or crypts. Patients commonly complain of an aching pain in the perineum. Mixed infections of aerobic and anaerobic bacteria are common causative agents. Smears of the aspirated material show numerous acute inflammatory cells and debris. ERUS-FNA with on-site evaluation provides a rapid diagnosis, and aspirated material can be sent for cultures.

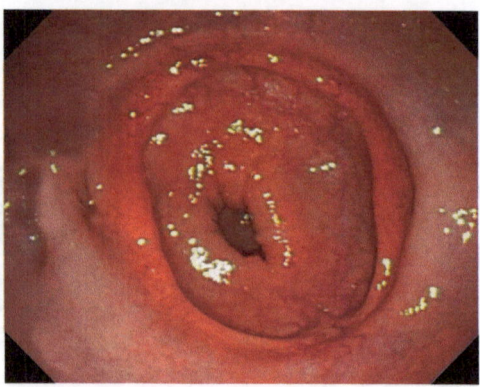

FIG. 6.28. Flexible sigmoidoscopy shows evidence of previous colonic re-section with patent anastomosis in the rectum. (Courtesy of Drs. Vikesh K. Singh and Joanna Law, The Johns Hopkins Hospital, Maryland, USA).

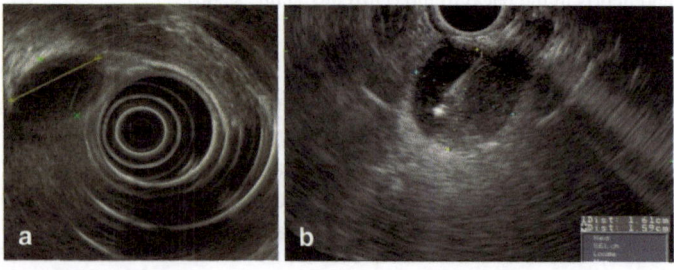

FIG. 6.29. a–b Radial ERUS (a) and ERUS-FNA (b) of a pararectal cyst. The cyst is anechoic with well-defined and uniform cyst wall. (a, b Courtesy of Drs. Vikesh K. Singh and Joanna Law, The Johns Hopkins Hospital, Maryland, USA).

ERUS may be useful for identifying and draining the abscess, which is the main line of treatment.

In summary, ERUS and ERUS-FNA are minimally invasive and highly accurate diagnostic and therapeutic modalities for evaluating colorectal masses, difficult to evaluate by other means. Material obtained by FNA is valuable as an adjunct to avoid more invasive procedures and guide patient management in a cost effective manner.

Further Reading

Baewer D, Adair C. Pathology of the anus. Gastrointestinal and liver pathology. Philadelphia: Elsevier Sounders; 2012. pp. 448–89.

Dahan H, Arrivé L, Wendum D, Docou lePH, Djouhri H, Tubiana JM. Retrorectal developmental cysts in adults: clinical and radiologic-histopathologic review, differential diagnosis, and treatment. Radiographics. 2001;21(3):575–84. Review.

Gallegos-Arreola MP1, Valencia-Rodríguez LE, Puebla-Pérez AM, Figuera LE, Zúñiga-González GM. The TP53 16-bp duplication polymorphism is enriched in endometriosis patients. Gynecol Obstet Invest. 2012;73(2):118–23. doi:10.1159/000330702. (Epub 2012 Feb 17).

Karlsson R, Aly M, Clements M, Zheng L, Adolfsson J, Xu J, Grönberg H, Wiklund F. A population-based assessment of germline HOXB13 G84E mutation and prostate cancer risk. Eur Urol. 2014;65(1):169–76. doi:10.1016/j.eururo.2012.07.027. (Epub 2012 Jul 20).

Kav T, Bayraktar Y. How useful is rectal endosonography in the staging of rectal cancer? World J Gastroenterol. 2010;16(6):691–7.

Maleki Z, Erozan Y, Geddes S, Li QK. Endorectal ultrasound-guided fine-needle aspiration: a useful diagnostic tool for perirectal and intraluminal lesions. Acta Cytol. 2013;57(1):9–18.

Miettinen M, Sarlomo-Rikala M, Sobin LH, Lasota J. Gastrointestinal stromal tumors and leiomyosarcomas in the colon: a clinicopathologic, immunohistochemical, and molecular genetic study of 44 cases. Am J Surg Pathol. 2000;24(10):1339–52.

Purysko AS, Coppa CP, Kalady MF, Pai RK, Leão Filho HM, Thupili CR, Remer EM. Benign and malignant tumors of the rectum and perirectal region. Abdom Imaging. 2014 Mar 25;39(4):824–52.

Rossi L, Palazzo L, et al. Can rectal endoscopic sonography be used to predict infiltration depth in patients with deep infiltrating endometriosis of the rectum? Ultrasound Obstet Gynecol. 2014;43(3):322–7.

Turaga KK, Kvols LK. Recent progress in the understanding, diagnosis, and treatment of gastroenteropancreatic neuroendocrine tumors. CA Cancer J Clin. 2011;61(2):113–32.

Vander NMR 3rd, Eloubeidi MA, Chen VK, Eltoum I, Jhala D, Jhala N, Syed S, Chhieng DC. Diagnosis of gastrointestinal tract lesions by endoscopic ultrasound-guided fine-needle aspiration biopsy. Cancer. 2004;102(3):157–63.

Index

R. H. Bardales (ed.), *Cytology of the Mediastinum and Gut Via Endoscopic* 151
Ultrasound-Guided Aspiration, Essentials in Cytopathology 25,
DOI 10.1007/978-3-319-12796-5,
© Springer International Publishing Switzerland 2015